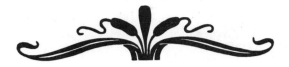

Nature's First Law:
The Raw-Food Diet

Contributing Authors:

Stephen Arlin
"Captain Wheatgrass"

Fouad Dini
"Raw Courage Vegetable Man"

David Wolfe
"Fats Avocado"

Nature's First Law:
The Raw-Food Diet

First Edition: April 20, 1996
Cover Photos: Marc Wolfe

Printed in North America by

Maul Brothers Publishing
PO Box 900202
San Diego, CA 92190

ISBN 0-9653533-0-3

Table Of Contents

Acknowledgment

This book is dedicated to the memory of Aterhov. For without his vast knowledge and inspiration, this work would not have been possible.

"Every step toward the Truth has had to be fought for at the expense of all that human hearts and human love hold dear."
— **Friedrich Nietzsche**

Preface

It is very difficult to explain something of this majesty and glory to indoctrinated and closed minds. However, it must be said that Nature's First Law has arrived just in the nick of time to salvage humanity and put it back on the course of evolution. We are troubadours of the truth. The truth we stand for encompasses the scientific facts and demonstrable realities of life. We have arrived to defend Nature.

The irrefutable truth of our information hits hard and gives no quarter. The truth always has enemies. Though it has invariably been opposed, it has inevitably prevailed. The medical, pharmaceutical, livestock, and cooked-food industries do not like what we are saying. It is dangerous to be right when everybody else is wrong.

We represent the very nature of Truth and we will continue to represent it in every manifestation. We proceed under the operative principle that any philosophy or religion that denies any of the Laws of Nature is false. It is in this light which we demonstrate that humanity has made fundamental errors which have all-encompassing ramifications.

Parts of this book have been published in past Nature's First Law newsletters. In those newsletters, which comprised brief summaries of our philosophical views on nutrition, we touched upon almost every important aspect of natural nutrition. Generally speaking, there is no need to enter into long-winded details in order to declare to the world the simple truth that the operations of cooking and refining are not only unnatural, harmful, and break the Laws of Nature, but they are the primary cause of all diseases. The most ignorant person can clearly perceive that, instead of freeing people from diseases, medical science (with its cooked foods and poisonous drugs) has lead humankind into a multitude of serious ailments, from which all undomesticated living creatures are immune.

After reading only a few lines on the subject, clear-sighted people awaken from their lethargic indifference and realize the full gravity of the situation. The vast majority of people, however, who are intoxicated by current medical theories, scientific misconceptions, and prejudiced by a host of other preconceived ideas often wish and, in fact, need further information on the subject. That is why, in this book, we have come forward with an entire philosophy of natural nutrition including detailed explanations on a number of crucial questions. By giving up cooked foods and poisonous drugs many sensible people all over the world have cured themselves of their long-standing illnesses and are now enjoying carefree lives filled with health and happiness.

When a new machine or instrument is invented, a few successful tests are deemed sufficient to confirm and prove the validity of that invention. Today thousands of healthy people throughout the world are living proof that raw-foodism saves humankind from the ruthless clutches of every disease on Earth. One might well have thought that this would have sufficed to arouse the scientific world from its sluggish apathy and convince everybody of the enormous benefits that raw-foodism brings for us all. But that is not the case.

Today, people, blinded by cooked-food addiction, organize international conferences to combat disease, pollution, and supposed world shortages of food. They deliver endless speeches on ridiculous subjects, while 90 percent of the real foods given to us by Nature are thoughtlessly destroyed by cooking and refining.

Our information appeals to humanity as a whole. Raw-foodism disposes of incalculable ailments and problems. Diseases, obesity, depression, pollution, etc. — all of these things are caused by the consumption of cooked food. If you are ill, consume exclusively raw plant food and your illness will wither away. If you are overweight, eating raw will restore your body to its natural weight. If you suffer from depression, eating raw will restore happiness and vitality. If you are an environmentalist, start by cleaning up your own body.

Our organization, Nature's First Law, is dedicated to bringing about a world in which disease, pollution, famine, and ignorance will be only memories of a dismal past.

Chapter 1

Our Realization

"If you shut up the truth and bury it under the ground, it will but grow, and gather to itself such explosive power that the day it bursts through, it will blow up everything in its way."
— **Emile Zola**

Raw plant food should be the only food eaten by human beings. Humanity's habit of eating cooked food must be abandoned in this world once and for all. This is the absolute command of Nature. The consumption of cooked food is the most unnatural savagery in the history of humankind. It is an atrocity that no one seems to be aware of and to which everybody falls an unconscious victim. What people eat deeply and radically affects the way they think, feel, and behave. It drastically affects the entire life process of planet Earth. No matter how strange the idea may seem to some, it is the absolute truth that humanity must accept. To most, the truth is stranger than fiction.

This truth became evident to these three authors when, after years of careful study and investigation, we became convinced that the deaths of our family members, friends, and pets were caused by unnatural nutrition. In turn, improper nourishment caused the premature degeneration of their cellular structures. All the medical examinations carried out to diagnose their specific diseases and all the drugs and medicines they were coerced to ingest also had a considerable share in bringing the tragedy to a head. Our family members, friends, and pets died of the gradual emaciation and wasting away of their internal organs caused by unnatural feeding and poisonous medicines.

We have been able to penetrate into the secrets of medical science and to observe its good and bad aspects. We have not been driven by the prospect of becoming doctors or by making any financial gains by lying. First, our incentive has been to do our best to help our families and friends achieve greater levels of health. And later, it has been the ardent desire to perpetuate the memory of those family members and friends who have passed away by being useful to humanity.

Another factor which has contributed to our better realization of the shortcomings of medical science is the entirely natural system by which we have carried out our studies. We have engaged in a rigorous regimen of self-education and objective truth-seeking, free from the encumbrance of an indoctrinating academic program. We have never become intoxicated by the exaggerated claims of progress made on behalf of medical science or by all the fanciful tales of the fabulous benefits derived from medicines. We have approached these questions with critical minds and have always laid greater stress on their shortcomings. Moreover, we have constantly kept in view the fact that, in spite of the existence of millions of doctors and a large number of Nobel Prize winners, human beings fall victim to various illnesses far more often than any other animal. Diseases like osteoporosis, diabetes, heart disease, and cancer are still increasing at an alarming rate, threatening to wipe humanity off the face of the Earth.

We have searched Nature, not libraries, for facts. Most people live their lives like machines, conforming to their society only to discover in the end that they had never really lived. We have learned to confront only the essential facts of life and see what Nature has to teach. Nature is the only teacher we have ever trusted.

Throughout our search we have always kept in mind two essential principles:

First, we have clearly understood that the belief in even one false principle is the beginning of all unwisdom and the end of all knowledge.

Second, we have completely grasped the fact that false knowledge is more dangerous than ignorance.

We have not wasted our time in memorizing the symptoms of diseases, the names and doses of medicines and those numerous complicated formulae that are seldom needed. We have never had the intention of taking examinations and obtaining degrees in medicine or nutrition.

The results of years of painstaking study and labor have been embodied in this work. As far as possible, we have devoted our time to the study of a great many branches of science and to the sources of these multifarious categories of knowledge.

We have drawn certain, essential, vital conclusions:

Cooked food is poison.

Cooked food is drug addiction.

Cooked food is the source of all disease...no exception.

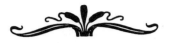

Chapter 2

Discovery Of Fire

"But Zeus was angered in his heart and hid the means to life because Prometheus with his crooked schemes had cheated him. This is why Zeus devised sorrows and troubles for men—he hid fire. But Prometheus, noble son of Iapetos, stole it back for man from Zeus, whose counsels are many. In the hollow of a fennel stalk he slipped it away, unnoticed by Zeus, who delights in thunder. So the cloud-gatherer in anger said to him: 'Son of Iapetos, there is none craftier than you, and you rejoice at tricking my wits and stealing the fire which will be a curse to you and to the generations that follow. The price for the stolen fire will be a gift of evil to charm the hearts of all men as they hug their own doom.'"
— Hesiod

Until the discovery of fire, along with the rest of the animal world, humans had evolved exclusively on natural, raw nourishment. But since the discovery of fire, without much reflection, human beings have put natural foodstuffs on the fire, destroyed their essential constituents, debased them, and then malnourished their bodies with them. What has resulted as a direct consequence of this activity are all the diseases that afflict humankind today.

The human is one of the most complicated organic machines ever constructed by the unceasing efforts of Nature. Homo sapien is the product of more than 1.5 billion years of animal evolution.

Simultaneously, with the construction of this living machine, Nature has incorporated the life-giving rays of the Sun to develop all the raw plant materials which are required to coordinate the billions of complex operations performed by the human organism each day. Moreover, Nature has placed those constituent raw materials in their complete and total perfection and harmony within each kernel of corn, each pulpy seed of the pomegranate, each grape, and every luscious melon. Each of these, and all other living foodstuffs, contain all the elements which are necessary to maintain, in perfect health, all the organic functions of the human body.

Try to picture for a moment the wonders that Nature performs. It really is beyond comprehension. People say they have never seen a miracle before: What then is the process that turns a blueberry into flesh and bone? As soon as that single berry is introduced into the alimentary canal, the organism softens it, breaks it down, and distributes it throughout the body. The countless substances that are concentrated in that berry move in all directions; each goes to perform its specific duty. Thus, the various nutritive elements in a blueberry perform upwards of six million different tasks and conduct the biological functions of the organism without the slightest flaw.

In contrast, the fire-processing of food has the effect of evaporating indispensable living water from plant foods and of rendering animal products inert so as to become palatable. And steaming is no better — it turns vegetables into inorganic sulfur deposits which are devoid of life and reek of some terrible, unnatural stench.

Fire is an equal opportunity destroyer. You cannot break down the cellulitic walls of vegetables (to make them more "digestible") without destroying the water-soaked nutrients contained within that fiber.

When you cook food above 38.9 degrees Celsius (102 degrees Fahrenheit), the enzyme metabolism begins to disrupt and break down. Nothing works without enzymes. Enzymes are the life catalyst behind every function the human body performs. That is why a fever is so dangerous. At 38.9 degrees Celsius (102 degrees Fahrenheit) you literally start to cook. On a cooked, enzymeless diet the body is forced to overwork its indigenous (or internal) enzymes to break down those unnatural materials. The body requires exogenous (or external enzymes) in the form of raw plant food.

All cooked foods damage the body — a little at a time. When a slice of bread is introduced into the body, the stomach aimlessly attacks the bread with acids and ptyalin. The dryness of the bread increases one's thirst inordinately. The bread is eventually broken down into a paste and passed into the intestines where some of its constituent parts pass through the intestinal villi. At best the cells derive some faulty nourishment from the whole process. Bread causes unnatural modes of existence and infamous crimes against Nature. The heart that feeds on raw, living wheat is as strong and powerful as the wheat field itself; whereas the heart that feeds on bread is as flimsy and pliable as the bread itself. It is no wonder people degenerate and expire at such a young age.

In the mechanical world, the slightest deviation from the details developed by an engineer for the smooth functioning of a machine, or a fault in the raw supplies specified to ensure its normal productivity, results in a corresponding breakdown in the machine. Similarly, the slightest alteration or degeneration of the raw materials prescribed by Nature to ensure the smooth functioning of the incredibly complicated human organism causes corresponding disorders within the organs of the body. These disorders appear in the form of diseases.

The multifarious methods employed by humanity in destroying or degenerating the fully balanced raw materials prescribed by Nature for the human organism are too vast to comprehend. For that purpose, "civilized" humanity has invented maniacal factories, furnaces, freezers, stoves, ovens, toasters, and kitchens. *Every degeneration in the quality of natural foodstuffs is categorically followed by a subsequent degeneration in the human organism.* "Cause and Effect" is the eternal law of human destiny. Natural nutrition guarantees the normal operation of the human organism, while unnatural nutrition is followed by an abnormal perturbation in its functions. The multiplicity of illnesses that presently afflict the world are the direct result of the vast, unchecked degeneration of natural foodstuffs.

Provided that all its needs are satisfied by the immutable Laws of Nature, the human organism, which is one of the most perfect organisms in the animal world, can live in excellent health for up to 150 years and beyond depending on each individual's genetic history and predisposition. Cooked and other denatured foods force human organs to work up to four or five times their normal capacity, thus exhausting them prematurely, while at the same time causing illnesses that shorten and degenerate the quality of human life.

In this present age of "scientific advance" humanity could easily rid itself of the loathsome diseases of civilization by complete abstinence from cooked food. Simultaneously, along with natural nutrition, people must make certain that all the other natural requirements of the body are met. These include: exercise, rest, clean air, deep breathing, sunshine on the skin, air bathing, abstinence from artificial heating, stretching, massage (being touched by others), intelligent thinking, and loving relationships.

Cooked food is poison.

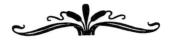

Chapter 3

Disease

"Doctors simply address the symptoms caused by the consumption of cooked, dead, or denatured foodstuffs."
— **Nature's First Law**

Diseases are not psychosomatic in origin as popular myth dictates — diseases are not created in the mind. Diseases are only psychosomatic in the sense that mental stress constricts the nerves and hampers the eliminative efforts of the body. It is the reaction to trapped poisons in the tissues of the body which creates diseases. The real cause of pathological conditions in the human organism, lies not in some externally originating invasion of the body by swarming masses of microbes, demons, evil spirits, bad luck, or other such exotic agents of causation, but in the internal reaction, in the form of trapped wastes and poisons, to the consumption of denatured, intoxicating beverages and foods. All diseases, degenerations, and chronic ailments in all plants and animals are caused by microscopic or macroscopic physical obstructions — anything which loosens, removes, and eliminates these obstructions from the organism gives health. In animals, the primary source of these obstructions is the food material coming in. For humans the problem is severe because cooked food is so lifeless, dehydrated, and damaging.

There are four basic types of disease:

1. A deficiency in the number of differentiated cells.

2. An insufficiency of the raw materials necessary for the functioning of the organs.

3. The presence of foreign bodies and parasitic cells in the organism.

4. A weakening in the resistance of the cells due to bacterial infection.

Raw-foodism mercilessly destroys all four of these sources and offers an absolute solution to the problem of disease.

Sources one and two are the direct nutritional ailments. Direct nutritional diseases are caused by a superabundance of certain unnatural constituents or a deficiency of natural foods. All chronic disorders and deficiency diseases fall into this category. These diseases develop slowly and secretly. So long as the disease has not entered its final stages, and the organs are still operating, people regard themselves as "healthy." Most of these disease types fit into familiar catagories, but in the event of a partial or mixed degree of unnatural foodstuffs and a deficiency of natural vitamins, coupled with the variation in human genetic weaknesses, the disease may appear in a form different from those described in medical books and thus it may be diagnosed as "rare" or "unique."

Sources three and four are the indirect nutritional ailments. Indirect digestive ailments are the "infectious" or "parasitic" diseases. Within the human organism lives an enormous variety of bacteria and microbes which, under normal circumstances, render useful service to the organism. The specialized or differentiated cells not only control and direct the "worker" cells but also the bacteria and microbes living in the system. However, through faulty nutrition, the specialized cells at last succumb to degeneration and emaciation. They become so weakened that by the Law of Survival, the bacteria and microbes get the upper hand, set themselves free from the control of those cells, rebel against their leaders, become pathogenic, and cause those infamous "infectious diseases." "Might is Right" remains an eternal, biological truth.

Sometimes, invading armies of assailing microbes or ingested parasites establish a hold upon the nutritionally emaciated body and cause their specific infections. Such invaders would have been met with impenetrable opposition and been crushed at once in a healthy organism.

The fear of microbes has so frightened people that, to escape them, they have taken recourse to the most dangerous measures only to achieve, in a greater ferocity, the result they sought most to avoid. The cooking of raw food and the unrestrained ingestion of laboratory invented chemicals in order to avoid microbes is perhaps the most fatal mistake of medical science. Humans cannot exterminate microbes from the Earth, nor should they want to. Microbes are found everywhere, even where life itself is most perilous. They will always exist. They can enter the human body through a multiplicity of channels. By cooking food, people weaken the bacterial resistance of both their "worker" and specialized cells. They then burn those natural antibiotics that are developed by Nature to control harmful microbes. Even cooked-food biologists would confirm that many vitamins, even some that have been almost entirely destroyed by the kitchen fire, still retain bactericidal properties.

A raw-foodist has no fear of bacteria, germs, or viruses, because s/he is protected against them by natural forces. Microbes cannot harm the fully developed and specialized (differentiated) cells. They spread their ravages on the weak, delicate, "civilized" cells.

Cooked food is poison.

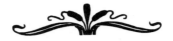

Chapter 4

Adaptation?

"Ponce de Leon wandered around looking for the Fountain of Youth and all the while his mare was grazing on it."
— **Nature's First Law**

Many cooked-foodists are inclined to believe that because people have fed on cooked food for thousands of years, the human race must have become adapted to it and would now suffer upon returning to a raw-food diet.

First of all, any major physiological adaptation encompassing all the digestive and supporting organs of the body involves epochs of change and mutation spanning millions of years. The period of 500,000 years, since the discovery of fire, is nothing in comparison with the 1,500,000,000 years during which humanity and its genetic forebears lived and developed exclusively on raw food.

Secondly, only within the past few thousand years have cooked foods comprised such a large percentage of the human diet. Indeed, this is for the most part due to the proliferation of technology and the growth of civilization.

Thirdly, only within the last few hundred years have such extremely degenerated foodstuffs such as white flour and refined sugar reached the masses.

Besides these facts, the most conclusive evidence that humans have not adapted to cooked food is the very existence of diseases themselves, which disappear "miraculously" and "spontaneously" once one returns to a raw-food diet.

If humans have "adapted" to eating cooked food, there should be no essential physiological differences between animals that feed exclusively on raw foods and human animals that feed on cooked foods. They should be biologically identical. Anyone who believes this should compare the blood of a human who feeds on cooked foods with that of a wild animal who feeds on living foods. Take note of the fact that humans suffer from hundreds of times more diseases than any other animal on Earth and that natural animals, living far from human civilization and denatured food, never suffer from any illnesses or diseases.

It is true that by the Laws of Evolution the human organism attempts to adapt itself to the food it receives, but not in the ways most people imagine, as we will show throughout this book.

Cooked food is poison.

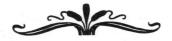

Chapter 5

Cooked Food: A Physio-Chemical Addiction

"Addiction conquers science and takes it into its talons."
— Aterhov

Many people naturally wonder why none of the numerous "learned" scientists and philosophers understand these simple Truths and why nobody has yet told humanity that eating cooked food is unnatural and dangerous. The reason is that all of humanity is addicted to cooked food and that addiction has blinded everybody. Nobody realizes that cooked-food eating is a vice. In fact, it is the most terrible vice of all. The danger of processing foods with heat and flame is a scientific fact that everyone wants to ignore because they are addicted to cooked food. Indeed, all science has really been a struggle in the human mind between humanity as it really is and humanity as people wish or hope it to be.

Cooked-food addiction encompasses not just a craving for one type of substance, but hundreds, even thousands, of substances. On top of this, short-sighted cooked-eaters see richness and excellence in the multiplicity of debased foodstuffs. It is that very multiplicity of debasements that gives rise to a multiplicity of harms. A true reflection of this hedonism can be seen in the large variety of illnesses that prevail in the world — especially in the "rich, developed" world.

Human beings become addicted to substances that contain poisons, such as tea, coffee, cooked marijuana, cooked tobacco, alcohol, cocaine, heroin, etc. Addictions promote and defend themselves.

The strong craving for those substances is stimulated by corresponding poisons collected in the human organism. Cooked foods contain a large variety of poisons which, in the course of time, accumulate in different parts of the body. They are deposited on the walls of the veins and the capillaries, between the joints, in the center of fat cells, and elsewhere.

The crack addict's craving for rock cocaine does not arise out of the normal physiological needs of the organism; it is created by a physio-chemical addiction. Similarly, the desire for cooked food is not a physiological need, but a physio-chemical addiction. It is the expression of impulses that are stimulated by the poisons and malformed cells thriving in the organism. It is the demand of diseases rooted in the body, the call of humanity's worst enemy.

That terrible vice is introduced into the body of every human being by her or his own mother when still an embryo via the umbilical cord and placenta. Once the child is born, the parents unwittingly continue this insane process. Even before a child has learned to talk, cooked-food addiction has already secured a physio-chemical hold on the organism. From that moment until the end of life, s/he regards cooked food as normal and natural and the craving for it, s/he mistakes for hunger.

Cooked food is poison.

Chapter 6

Cooked Food Is Not Nourishment

"I am repelled by this mad sorcery.
I shall get well, you promise me,
In this chaotic craziness?
Shall I demand an old crone's remedy?
Will this absurd swill-cookery
Charm thirty winters off my back?
Woes me, if there's naught better you can find!
For now my hope already disappears.
Has Nature not, has not some noble mind,
Discovered somewhere any elixirs."
— Johann Wolfgang von Goethe, *Faust*

When cooked-foodists feed exclusively on natural foodstuffs such as fruits, vegetables, herbs, honey, or wheatgrass they have met the natural demands of their organism and are, at that moment, completely satiated. However, instead of feeling lighter and more happy, cooked-food addicts become edgy and irritated. They still behave as if they had eaten nothing at all and feel a great demand for foods such as a dish of "enriching" pasta and white rice or grilled steak and mashed potatoes. In their opinion the reason for their continuous hunger lies in the absurd notion that raw foods must be of low nutritional value and are not complete and "heavy" enough for "real" food. This is a terrible misconception. There is nothing healthy or natural about the "full and satisfied" feeling that cooked-foodists feel after a meal. Such a condition is nothing more than an addictive fix. A paralyzed stomach is the very hallmark of cooked-food addiction.

In reality, the physiological demand for cooked food is not caused by hunger. It is caused by the movement of poisons which are suddenly in "danger" of being purged out of the system. It is the body's cry to remain clogged. It is the cry of disease and addiction that lies sprawled like a demon and demands new poisons with which to continue the erosion of the Life-force. *The valiant, strong-willed raw-foodist hears that cry in all its vehemence, but ignores it with every bit of might and does not make one concession to it.*

So long as there are any diseased cells in the human organism, there exists a strong craving for cooked food. But once the body is cleansed of its diseased cells, even the sight of cooked food fills the raw-foodist with displeasure. The stronger the feeling of "hunger," the deeper and graver the disease. Essentially, the desire for cooked food is a desire for disease. The persistence of that desire signifies the persistence of disease. In order to subdue and annihilate disease, it is necessary to starve malformed cells by fasting and eating only raw foods.

Raw plant foods are both nutritious and fully balanced. The cells of humanity have suffered for millennia due to their absence. The capacities of the human digestive organs fully correspond to their composition, especially the composition of fruit. That is why the stomach gladly welcomes these foodstuffs, softens them quickly, and passes them through the pyloric valve into the intestines without delay. Correspondingly, the cells, weakened and emaciated as they are with improper nutrients, avidly absorb those valuable substances and repeatedly demand more and more of them.

On a diet of raw plant foods, the diseased cells heal, the emaciated ones recuperate, the inactives regain their vitality. The fat cells, on the other hand, begin to shrink as toxins are discharged. The accumulation of poisons gradually disappears and superfluous dead water flows out of the body and is replaced by living plant fluids. Even negative and self-destructive emotions are purged from the system.

Eventually, normal, active cells take the place of those sluggish cells which were fattened with indolence and inaction. A quick loss in excess body weight is a sure sign of regained health and vigor. In fact, when one reaches her or his lowest weight, that is the denouement of the body's cleansing activity.

After that, the body's weight will increase until one has reached her or his ideal body proportions.

Additionally, no amount of raw food is ever fattening. The idea that bananas, coconuts, and avocados are fattening is not based on fact, it is just part of the elaborate cooked-food mythology.

These facts should fill the hearts of people with joy and happiness. Raw nutrients spread throughout the body, relax the organs, and grant health, strength, vigor, long life, and success. For most, it will be the first time in their entire life that they are able to live in comfort and ease.

A raw-food diet only provides advantages. Even when one consumes a massive amount of raw plant food, the body does not rebel, but simply derives exactly what it needs and expels the remaining material through the normal channels. Thus a raw-foodist's stomach is always light, while her or his intestines and blood are consistently loaded with fully-balanced nutrients.

But, if at any time one returns to eating even just a few morsels of cooked food the trouble begins anew. The stomach will react harshly to those strange and unwanted substances. In spite of the pleasure that the palate may feel, those cooked morsels will sit in the stomach for many hours; they will act as a plug in the intestines, backing up the body's "sewage" system; and they will be noticeable when expelled with the feces. Ignorantly, cooked-foodists are quite content and happy with that unnatural condition, because their base passions have been satisfied and their stomach is now "full." The person who realizes the value of eating raw dreads that condition. Raw-foodists fully grasp the fact that only raw plant food nourishes the body, while dead, cooked corpses and fired plant foods are the sources of unnatural behaviors and diseases.

Cooked food is poison.

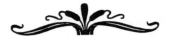

Chapter 7

True Body / False Body

*"I am sure that human beings have two distinct entities—
a good self and an evil self. My task is to use my
body for my experiment and try to extract my 'evil' self."*
— **Robert Louis Stevenson,** *Dr. Jeckyl and Mr. Hyde*

The addicted consumer of cooked food is actually a combination of two entities in one; s/he has two bodies. The first one is the "true body," the true human, which has been called into being by means of natural nourishment and is still sustained by natural nutrition. The second one is the mutant "false body," which has been brought into existence by means of unnatural, cooked, artificial food and continues to exist on unnatural nutrition alone.

All those cells in the human body that, being healthy, specialized, and active, maintain life and keep human beings on their feet are constructed, nourished, operated, and replaced entirely by natural foodstuffs. Those are the cells that give endurance to the muscles, regulate the constrictions of the heart, transmit the nerve impulses of the brain to the body, and produce glandular secretions.

Beside these highly developed cells there are other cells that bear some superficial resemblance to normal cells except that they have not evolved beyond elementary stages. They lack the necessary organelles and mechanisms for specialized functions and are generally degenerated and diseased. These cells are born, bred, and multiplied entirely at the expense of unnatural and debased food.

The false body is not composed of only degenerated cells, but also a plethora of fluids, fats, concretions, salts, poisons, and other harmful substances, which have penetrated and spread into all the cavities and tissues of the true body. *Every illness, without exception, is called into being in the cells of the false body.*

In the organism of a cooked-food addict the true body occupies very little space. Even in the most emaciated and thinnest individuals a considerable proportion of the body consists of inactive, dormant, and degenerated cells.

Each gland or organ needs a certain number of active and specialized cells. As soon as the requisite complement of such cells is formed, the construction of additional cells in the given organ stops, otherwise it would grow to an inordinate size. Now, because active cells are called into being only through natural nourishment, the organ is obliged to offset the resulting deficiency and keep its size within reasonable limits by amassing a certain number of inactive cells produced from cooked food. Studies done by cytologists show that, in addition to indolent cells, various multinucleated giant cells (polykaryocytes), uninucleated over-sized cells (megakaryocytes) and other types of degenerated cells are found in the human body. Such cells are always present in the tissues of cooked-foodists.

Researchers who see these and other aberrations in the organs of all cooked-food addicts regard them as "normal" or "natural" occurrences. Such useless and parasitic cells abound in all the organs and systems of a cooked-food addict, even in the bones, brain, nervous system, and teeth. The basis of all research experimentation, and "facts" pertaining to medical science today are conducted on false body systems and organs. *We must conclude that all science and research that is founded on such debased subject matter is moot and quite meaningless.*

Nevertheless, some people are able to struggle against unnatural diets for a certain period of time. Indeed, the organism tries its best to prevent the formation of the false body by diminished appetite (anorexia nervosa), stomach disorders, nausea, vomiting (bulemia), insomnia, headaches, and other similar means. Short-sighted people regard such precautionary symptoms as signs of some debility of the organism, so instead of stopping the consumption of unnatural materials, they encourage their increased use in order to "nourish and strengthen" the individual. And while under the continual assaults of "nutritious" foods the long drawn-out struggle comes to a tragic end with the defeat of the true body. The organism is forced to abandon its tenacious resistance and "adapt" itself to those unnatural foodstuffs. This is the signal for the birth of the false body, which soon begins to devour like a creeping mold and grow irresistibly. Yet short-sighted people regard this growth as a sure sign of recuperation.

In the course of many generations that resistance has become weaker. Today the stage has been reached when almost all children are born with two bodies. Such children begin to develop a false body even before they come into the world. What chance does an in-utero child have when its mother feeds exclusively on denatured foods? Humanity is breeding a chemical youth.

You can see the false body everywhere you turn: on the buttocks and legs of women, on the fat cheeks of children, on the hulking, slobbing bellies and triple-chins of men, and else-where. The false body deforms the pristine figures of young ladies in the prime of their lives. It deprives "middle-aged" people of their capacity to work. In extreme circumstances, it keeps people from carrying out the most simple of activities: walking, sitting, bending over, etc.

In advanced stages, the false body penetrates into the heart, kidneys, blood vessels, glands, and various tissues and paralyzes their movements. Quite literally, it takes the true body into its clutches and gradually squeezes and strangles it.

When a cooked-food addict satisfies her or his hunger by consuming some fruit, it means that at that given moment the true body is fully satiated and has no further desire for food. But the false body has received no share of the natural food at all, so it demands its own special food now. What makes matters particularly unfortunate is the fact that it expresses its strange desires through the mouth of the true body. The voracious craving for cooked food is the urge of that monster and has no connection whatsoever with the demands of the true body. That craving changes into gluttony at the moment when the two brutish passions, addiction and unnatural desires, join forces.

It is here that the true body, without any thought or reflection, performs a most demented task. It toils incessantly day after day, earns money with great pain and trouble. Then, with even more hardship and trouble, it turns the natural foods (that it has bought with its hard-earned money) into harmful substances. The true body introduces them into its body through its own mouth, digests them in its alimentary canal, and absorbs them into its bloodstream. The true body delivers them to that monster, its fiercest enemy, whom it rears and nurtures in its own bosom and whose abominable body it continually carries about on its weakly muscles.

Here we must ask biologists, who eulogize proteins and pin false hopes on the supposed potency of artificial vitamins, if they pity those wo/men who wobble and totter as they trudge along the street, barely able to drag forth the enormous weight of the false body on their frail legs. Where is the conscience and reason of those people? Do those masses of useless fat and flesh not give them any food for thought? After all, corpulence is the unnatural byproduct of their "fully-balanced" animal proteins and "digestible" bread. Just try to deprive those fat people of their bread and meat, and feed them for a time by the most elementary Laws of Nature, then notice how those masses melt and disappear within a few months. When you consider how easily you can get rid of those superfluous heaps of flesh and achieve a complete recovery by the most simple and natural methods, you may well wonder why people of high academic distinction have recourse to a surplus of dangerous and senseless techniques, without any prospect of success.

Cooked food is poison.

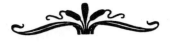

Chapter 8

Overworked Organs

*"Humans dig their graves with their own teeth
and die more by those fated instruments
than the weapons of their enemies."*
— **Thomas Moffett**

All human organs maintain a reserve of stored energy. Under natural conditions they work at twenty percent of their capacity, keeping the remaining eighty percent of that potential for use in the event of an emergency or just for the latter years of life. Thus, people who eat uncooked, natural foods never overload or fatigue their digestive organs.

However, people who binge on cooked foods, filling their stomachs with meats, corrosive salts, irritating spices, refined sugars, loathsome breads, pastas, and grotesque soups force their digestive organs to expend their reserve energies. Sometimes, the organs are so overworked they must quickly expel the food material either through the mouth (vomit) or intestines (diarrhea). Surprisingly enough, such nauseating acts are not considered strange by cooked-eaters, but are merely due to the "flu" or a "virus."

Natural foods, especially fruits, do not remain in the digestive organs for more than a few hours and, whether wholly digested or not, leave the body by normal channels. Cooked foods, especially those derived from animals, linger in the alimentary canal for three or four days, sometimes for weeks. The body labors to the point of exhaustion to eliminate these materials.

It is well known that immediately after an animal's death, its cells begin to decompose releasing a variety of toxins. It is no wonder that after remaining in the human abdomen for three days at a temperature of 37 degrees Celsius (98.6 degrees Fahrenheit) animal products are completely converted into poisons. Sometimes this process advances to such an extent that only after they have ravaged the walls of the intestines and have become mixed with considerable quantities of mucus, pus, and blood do they succeed in leaving the organism. Some "learned" doctors typically recommend the use of table salt in order to prevent such a putrefaction; they wish to convert the human bowels into a barrel of salted meat. Others recommend the use of adult diapers.

Overloading the digestive organs also causes other ancillary organs such as the liver, heart, and kidneys to work overtime. The additional work performed by these organs fatigues them prematurely. It is not surprising, therefore, that one's life-span is shortened by the same degree to which the organs are overworked. By feeding on useless, harmful, and poisonous substances cooked-food addicts gratify their passions, paralyze their stomachs, and create the illusion of being satisfied. In reality, however, the cells are moaning with hunger due to a lack of essential nutrients. A raw-foodist's stomach is always at rest because it is usually empty; at the same time the raw-foodist's body is fully biologically satisfied.

Cooked-foodists live on the work of one fifth of their organs, and yet, as long as they are able to stand on two feet, they regard themselves as healthy. Worse still, the danger of being deprived of those last functional cells hangs over them like a teetering boulder, especially when they have had a big holiday meal (e.g., Thanksgiving dinner with their close friends, family, etc.).

In the opinion of cooked-foodists, one must eat well-balanced meals in order to maintain good health. In their view, an empty stomach means a hungry body. They do not realize that a paralyzed stomach equals a sick body. The stomach expends an enormous amount of energy in order to pass unnatural foods into the small intestine.

A raw-foodist's stomach is always empty or it is so light that s/he does not feel anything there. A raw-foodist occasionally feels a fullness in the bowels because that is where the food s/he has eaten is immediately transferred. Even excess food does not lie in a raw stomach for long; it quickly passes into the intestines and, digested or undigested, leaves the body without causing the least harm to the organism.

If a raw-foodist consumes only one type of food per meal, no gases are ever generated in the stomach and colons. If an excessive amount of food (eaten in various combinations) is consumed, gases may be generated, but they leave the body by the normal route. Each food ferments at a slightly different rate; each food has its peculiar enzymes. Conflicting fermentation rates and enzymatic clashes cause flatulence.

Raw-foodists see the difference between the two systems of nutrition all the more clearly when they try to return to their former eating habits after a few months of abstinence. It is then that they wonder how they could ever have dragged on such a sickly and miserable existence and have regarded that disgusting mode of life as normal.

Cooked-food addicts cannot regard themselves as healthy. The foundation of their ill-health has been laid by their own mothers, even before they were born. Their organs are weak and every moment they live in danger of exhausting their last energy reserves. After reading these lines, those who value their health must make a firm decision to ward off that danger and repair, as fully as possible, the damage already done to their bodies. In particular, those people who suffer from obesity, smoking addictions, and high-blood pressure should not hesitate for a moment; their lives hang by a thread. They must not allow the ominous word "unexpected" to appear in the next day's obituaries. That word is a most striking example of "civilized" humanity's preposterous ignorance.

Cooked food is poison.

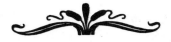

Chapter 9

Living Plant Cells

"The thin layer of soil that forms a patchy covering over the continents controls our own existence and that of every other animal on the land. Without soil, land plants as we know them could not grow, and without plants no animal could survive."
— **Rachel Carson**

All fully balanced foodstuffs consist of living cells. Plants extracted from the Earth and fruits plucked from a tree continue to live a long time once picked. A rosebud continues to bloom in a vase, an orange continues to ripen in a basket. But the cells of killed animals (and of mucous products or milks) die quickly, often within a few hours, that is why true carnivores eat their food when it is freshly killed, initially devouring the bowels and enzymatic organs, which decompose rapidly. Disintegrating cells eventually become poisonous, but cooking turns them into some kind of disgusting abomination. To regard dead animal proteins as superior to living vegetable proteins is an unfortunate error of judgment, a manifest proof of the short-sightedness of meat-worshipping parents, biologists, and nutritionists. If the flesh of herbivorous animals was such a tremendous source of "well-balanced" proteins then the carnivores that feed upon them should themselves have the most nutritious flesh of all; but even the most seasoned meat addict knows full well the poisonous character of such flesh and does not dare feed on it. Carnivores are scavengers. They are only able to take down the weakest members of herds consisting of thousands of animals.

Those doctors, biologists, and dietitians who are urged by their personal predilections to look for special advantages in meat by supposedly uncovering "indispensable" amino acids and other such nonsense have somehow overlooked the fact that those amino acids are formed from the commonest grasses consumed by animals. *By what rule of science has the gorilla or the orangutan the capacity to draw amino acids from plant foods and synthesize proteins to form their flesh, but humans somehow lack the capacity to do so?*

The whole science of nutrition may be summarized in two simple points:

1. Human nourishment must consist entirely of living plant cells. Only those foods that consist of living cells have all the qualities necessary to satisfy the demands of the human body. The most evolved creatures are the plant eaters. The most evolved plants foods are the fruits. The most advanced fruit eater is Homo sapien. Humans are biological frugivores. Humans are not omnivorous, carnivorous, nor necrophagus animals. The habit of eating long-dead, once-frozen, and inevitably cooked animal flesh is totally unnatural. Humans have no innate desires to eat moths out of the air (as a dog might) or to take down animals in the wild and tear them to pieces, whilst consuming their bloody flesh, bones and all. How long would you continue to eat flesh if you had to make your own kills?

2. The most perfect and highly nourishing plant foods are the fruits, especially the melons, apples, citrus, berries, bananas, avocados, peppers, chiles, and tomatoes. Avocados and bananas are not fattening — that is a total myth. These three authors lost a combined 180 pounds, while increasing our strength, by eating massive amounts of avocados which are indigenous and grow abundantly in our native Southern California. We find it quite amusing when someone who eats 90 percent cooked food won't eat avocados because they are "fattening." Raw fruits and vegetables are never harmful. Macrobioticists believe that night-shade plants are dangerous; they are, but only when cooked. These cooked-food morons similarly attack the sugar content of fruit. Fruit sugars are perfectly balanced and can never overburden the body, in fact the brain uses glucose exclusively for fuel — unnatural sugars are always harmful.

After understanding these two points the raw-foodist should bear in mind three goals:

1. Food should be eaten as freshly picked as possible.

2. Whenever possible, one should eat indigenous food. The plant life associated with any locale exerts life-giving forces which shape the body and character of all the creatures living thereon. This force weaves the animals to the land and the land to the animals.

3. Only one type of food should be eaten at a time. In Nature you would not find an apricot tree next to a mango tree, next to a pear tree, next to a grape vine, next to a watermelon patch; that is why you should never eat a mixed fruit salad.

By eating cooked food humans destroy their alimentary instincts and condemn themselves to an unnatural existence. Humans enjoy perfect health when they feed exclusively on raw plant foodstuffs, and become ill to the extent that they consume cooked, dead, and denatured food, eventually dying miserably when they subsist exclusively on such a diet.

Cooked food is poison.

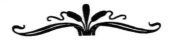

Chapter 10

Short-Sightedness

*"Decadence can find agents only
when it wears the mask of progress."*
— **Bernard Shaw**

The two greatest human flaws are short-sightedness and the unwillingness to take responsibility for one's own actions. People close their eyes to those harms that appear small and do not care to foresee the serious consequences that eventually arise from seemingly negligible causes.

For example: cooked meals, especially meat dishes, are full of toxins. Nobody takes any notice of the chronic poisoning that continuously, yet imperceptibly, goes on all the time. Even when, as a result of such poisoning, the heart, pancreas, liver, or kidneys are damaged, the condition is attributed to "unknown causes!" When the poisoning is more serious, it is regarded as terminal cancer. Only when the condition is severe and death is imminent do people finally contemplate taking action to correct the situation. Even then, due to the ocean of lies that fills the media, they inevitably choose the wrong course. How many lives are sacrificed due to ignorance?

The future is not a place you go, it is a place you create by the actions you take every day. People do not see the filth that passes into their arteries and veins through the foods they habitually eat. The human mouth is not a garbage can. Unnatural substances accumulate layer upon layer on the walls of blood vessels and arteries, narrowing their passages and one day "suddenly" stop the blood's circulation. Short-sighted people regard this occurrence as "unexpected." It wasn't the final straw which broke the camel's back; it was the accumulation of six million straws which led to the final collapse.

Every organ has billions of cells all working in concert. When the nourishment forced upon those cells lacks certain essential constituents, the cells begin to lose their vitality, and the organs lose their harmony. Energy reserves are called upon to maintain an organic balance. But so long as the organ somehow carries on its functions, short-sighted people do not see the warning signs. When the organ at last begins to lag behind, they lay the blame on unseen sources, and seek comfort in artificial medicines. It is impossible for a little (p)ill (a dose of poison) to ever replace the nutritive constituents of foodstuffs that have been burned over the fire. Medicines can never return those disabled cells to their lost capacity.

Nature dictates that if the power to fight for one's own health is no longer present, the right to live in this world of struggle ends. All people, no matter what their stations in life, are the sole possessors of their own body. They are the only ones responsible for that miraculous living ocean. If a person desires health s/he must take responsibility and develop a long-term plan based on the principles of natural nutrition or, more specifically, raw-foodism. *There simply is no other way.*

In the opinion of short-sighted, "civilized" humanity, eating raw is tantamount to a return to the primitive life of prehistoric humans. In point of fact there is no greater disgrace to human society than the operations of cooking and refining. The raw-foodist merely foregoes the miseries caused by the so-called "diseases of civilization" and refuses to promote the advances of technology towards unnatural ends. We are not against technology. We *are against* its application when no thought has been given to consequences. When a child first plays with fire s/he inevitably gets burned and thereafter remains cautious. The raw-foodist does not forgo the convenience of telephones, computer systems and electronic bulletin boards, traveling by air, land, and sea, or many of the other facets of technological living.

All of humanity has unwittingly accepted a Faustian bargain: a short-term pleasure at the expense of a long-term tragedy.

For countless millennia people have been so addicted, diseased, and ignorant that they have always regarded eating cooked meals as a natural procedure. Now, when for the first time they hear about raw-foodism, they think of it as something strange and curious, whereas in reality it is precisely the process of unwittingly consuming 1,000 cooked meals a year that is most unnatural, strange, and curious and which will undoubtedly be recorded in the annals of time as the greatest folly ever committed by Homo sapiens.

Cooked food is poison.

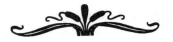

Chapter 11

Obesity

*"With such a great emphasis placed on
cleanliness in society, it is a wonder so few people
are concerned about the problem of internal filth."*
— Ann Wigmore

In the struggle to resist an unnatural diet, the human body "adapts" by making various complaints known, such as a loss of appetite, bad breath, rashes, indigestion, gastritis, ulcerative conditions, colitis, bulemia, and so on. All these are the outward manifestations of the internal struggle of the organism to use every means at its disposal to neutralize the harmful effects of an unnatural diet and purge poisonous substances from the body produced by it.

Cooked food eventually lands people in the most terrible of all places: a hospital. There, as a patient, one is "strengthened" by "wholesome, nutritious" meals along with medicines while doctors perform a myriad of tests to find out "what is wrong." This continues on, time and time again, until the day when the patient's body finally yields. The individual either bids farewell to life or begins to feel an increased appetite. The patient begins to put on weight and "to regain her or his health and strength." In other words, on that day the human organism, in abandoning its struggle, "adapts" itself to an unnatural diet and hence the foundation is laid for a disease of both mind and body — obesity. Nothing is more unnatural than a fat human being.

Subdued by the pressure of an unnatural diet, the body is forced to accommodate itself by admitting into the organism accumulations of various harmful substances. Deposits are then formed of fats, uric acid, cholesterol, inorganic salt, stale water, tumors, inactive and parasitic cells, multinucleated giant cells (polykaryocytes), cells with oversized nuclei (megakaryocytes), etc. Sometimes these deformed cells attain several hundred times the size of normal cells, but they lack the capacity to do any useful work.

All those abominations accumulate in the body to create the illusion of health and strength, while in actuality, the organism is gradually wasting away. Those "stout, robust, and jolly" men with bulging paunches, thick fat arms, large bellies, and over-hanging layers of fat are really skeletons covered with skin. Each of them has loaded their weak and debased muscles with a mass of fat acting as a repository for all the poisons they have ingested. But, strange to say, such people continually boast of their health, vigor, and strength. They are very proud of their puffed up musculature and their stoutness and defend these vigorously lest they should lose a gram of their cherished weight. These are the same people who "have never been sick a day in their whole life" but suddenly drop dead at age 45 from heart disease or colon cancer.

What happens when commercial interests and ill-advised doctors develop methods of reducing obesity? They plan an all encompassing restriction in the daily intake of food. Their lists of forbidden foods include such essential and highly-nutritive items as avocados, bananas, tomatoes, and honey. They reduce weight at the price of weakening the individual. Thus they seriously impair the individual's health. In such cases, the false body loses some of its superfluous fuel, but by any restriction of natural foods, the normal cells are deprived of some extremely essential nutrients. It follows then that the false body stays firm in its place, while the true body is emaciated all the more.

The thoughtless limitation of some arbitrary "calorie" intake has two contrary effects on the organism. On the one hand, the restricted consumption of degenerated foods inhibits the formation of disease and cancer, while on the other hand, the reduced intake of natural foods interferes with the normal activity of the organs. Medical science is full of such deplorable contra-dictions.

Eating raw bankrupts all the complex theories as to why and how people become fat.

Out of roast beef, bread, macaroni, wine, yogurt, soda, margarine, etc. are produced incapable, parasitic cells of a quite simple structure, under the weight of which the cooked-food addict stoops. Research scientists can easily prove by means of past literature that several hundred years ago human indispositions were mostly accompanied with excessive thinness. Society in that era was for the most part closer to Nature and unnatural foods were not so readily available. In those days humans also had a greater power of resistance; the human body was better able to withstand unnatural foodstuffs and to prevent the introduction of inordinate quantities of such substances by loss of appetite, diarrhea, vomiting, and other such means. However, in the course of time, human beings have yielded to an unceasing plumpness which appears in the "cute" faces of fat babies and grows worse with time. Today thinness is less common and the "rich, developed" world is filled with disgusting, unnatural corpulence.

Today many children are born with a terrible burden of worthless and inactive cells. Their parents are proud of their plump children with their chubby faces. Sometimes this plumpness is of such enormous dimensions that it terrifies those who understand its true nature. Yet foolish people represent those monstrosities, flaunted as "pictures of health" on the packages of denatured, cooked baby food, as sure signs of good health.

Cooked food is poison.

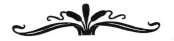

Chapter 12

Cancer

"You only get cancer if a cell
grows abnormally, not if it dies. "
— **Dr. Peter Duesberg**

The nutritive constituents of food that are essential for the intricate and specialized functions of the cells are easily destroyed by heat and flame. The foods that cooked-foodists consider "nutritious" lack essential elements. At the same time they have an abundant supply of dehydrated muscle proteins, animal fats, and dead carbohydrates, several times in excess of anything which a normal functioning cell can handle. A toxic, oxygen-poor environment is created within the organism.

Being continually deprived of oxygen and those nutritive elements that are essential for the performance of their higher functions, the cells typically do not attain their full development and specialization. If any cells do attain full development, they tend to prematurely lose their faculty of performing useful functions.

The human organism makes great efforts to keep the inordinate increase of parasitic and useless cells under control. The organism distributes them over all the free parts of the body: at the upper and lower extremities, underneath the chin, under the skin of the belly and the hips, and elsewhere.

After years of privation and endurance there comes a day when one of the billions of cells, genetically damaged and deprived of its remaining capabilities, is finally freed from the mechanisms that limit the growth of the cells. It then separates itself from life within the cellular community, becomes autonomous, and avariciously multiplies. Those "freed" cells devour the materials that have been rejected by the cells of the body as

greatly in excess of their needs, and which float in the inter-
cellular fluids. These materials are mostly the cooked proteins
— especially the cooked animal proteins. The proteins, of course,
are the food element most praised by the masses (especially
dietitians, doctors, nutritionists, etc.).

Though the body tries desperately to contain these primitive cells in tumorous formations, the uncontrolled, autonomous
cells continue to grow at an alarming speed. Because of the
flexibility of the organism the body often succeeds, at least for
a time, in keeping groups of those cells enveloped at one spot
and prevents them from spreading. The resulting growth is then
called a "benign neoplasm" or a "benign tumor." This is
distinguished from that growth which branches off freely to the
different parts of the body in order to thrive on proteins, and
which is known as a "malignant neoplasm." Heedless and
defiant, malignant cells multiply in a disorderly manner to form
an amorphous mass, a new living creature, which in the course
of its growth subdues and destroys everything in its surroundings
and at last one fine day fells that wonderful edifice, the human
organism. The name of that new creature is cancer. It is the true
offspring of cooked food; the living proof of how the cells have
evolved and "adapted" to the structure of those "nutritious"
foods people consume.

Cytologists have carried out an immense amount of research
in order to discover differences between the structures of normal
cells and those of cancer cells. They have found that cancer cells
are of a basic structure, lacking useful capability and differen-
tiation. Their only purpose is to devour dead proteins, typically
of animal origin, and multiply. As we have demonstrated, the
cells of the false body possess exactly the same qualities. There
is only a degree of difference between the cells of the false body
and cancer cells. Due to the flexibility of the organism the true
body is able to control the false cells for a long period of time.
The true body spreads the false cells among the free expanses of
the organism; it fills the empty cavities with them; disposes them
in the subcutaneous layers; it mixes them with the normal cells.
In this way the sensitive organs of the body are protected from
their pressure.

It is plain for everyone to see the enormous mass of the false body which often reaches a weight of fifty to sixty kilograms (110 to 130 lbs.). If even a kilogram of that mass were directly placed in any gland or organ, the activity of the given gland or organ would be paralyzed under the resulting pressure. It is precisely in this way that cancer puts an end to life.

The cells of the false body, like those of cancer, have been artificially conjured up by chefs and cooks. By its defensive efforts the true body is not able to completely assimilate the enormous quantities of unnatural substances entering the body due to addiction. In order to consume freely those excessive masses of food, the cells of the false body strive to obtain independence. They yearn to settle in any toxic location and fully gorge themselves. When a few succeed in their efforts, they begin to rapidly devour the excess foods proffered to them by their greedy host. Thus beginning with one or two insignificant cells, there comes into being that creature which keeps all of humanity in the clutches of its deadly terror.

In order to explain the occurrence of cancer, scientists have listed a thousand carcinogenic agents, which, with the exception of dietary factors, have not the least connection with the basic causes of carcinogenesis.

The power of cancer is found in baked, cooked, debased, degenerated, and denatured foods which enter the body by the command of the organism for its own ultimate demise. Cancer is the living proof of the extreme degeneration of cells and the inevitable result of unnatural nutrition.

As with all other diseases, the cause of cancer is quite easily explainable in light of the Laws of Nature. It is truly amazing that the cure to cancer and other diseases has been found but people are afraid to hear it!

Far-sighted people, who have the insight to occupy their minds with fundamental concerns, cannot help but wonder why research scientists waste so much time, energy, and money questioning obvious, demonstrable facts. During their investigations, scientists come face to face with the real causes of cancer. They hold the irrefutable proofs in their hands. They even confirm them.

But whenever the question of changing the prevailing dietary system comes up for deliberation, they close their cowardly eyes. They do not want to admit to themselves that their own feeding habits are unnatural. They would rather fool themselves and everyone else. Their own addictions thwart the scientific facts. They do not wish to criticize their bread which for all of humanity's disgusting religious and superstitious history has been regarded with such sanctity.

Any cytologist can tell you that cancer is brought into existence by abnormally grown cells that are devoid of specialized structures and operational capabilities. However in their view, all the cells of so-called "healthy" people — even though they are the product of unnatural nutrition — are primarily fully developed and perfect cells that are later deprived of their normal attributes through the influence of carcinogenic agents. They claim that the absence of proper mechanisms within the living machine or defects in its organic operation are connected with every causal factor. They do not see the defects in the building materials supplied to each cell. They do not want to see that the organs of all cooked-foodists are permanently inundated with billions of cells that have lost their proper structures and functions.

In spite of the paucity of their knowledge, research scientists ignore Nature's calculations. They induce people to believe, that by their own calculations, they can determine the exact qualitative and quantitative requirements of the cells. They even concoct various substances in their factories and offer them to the people of the world. We have trouble deciding whether this situation is laughable or deplorable.

Considerable evidence has been collected by research scientists to show that dietary restrictions of cooked food limit the incidence and growth of cancer. During the Gotterdammerung (the two world wars), under the severe food rationing in Austria, Germany, Russia, Britain, and Poland, cancer deaths declined dramatically.

Periods of war are very strange because they create a situation where a young individual's life may end abruptly or an elderly individual's life may be extended by cooked-food privations. When Norway was occupied by the Germans during the second world war, the Norwegian government was forced to sharply reduce the availability of dead animals to its citizens. Of course, the death rate from circulatory diseases dropped drastically. After the war, the Norwegians returned to their former diet — their death rates rose accordingly.

Among wild animals in Nature, cancer is unknown. After subjecting captive monkeys to degenerated foods for extended periods of time, however, cancer makes its appearance. Only those animals that have not reached the cooked hands of humanity are safe.

The types of food they give to experimental mice, the highly purified materials, such as casein (from pasteurized cow's milk), dead starch, cooked vegetable oil, synthetic vitamins, hormones, and salts are the cause of cancer in those mice. The mixture of these substances is misnamed a "normal diet" by researchers. They collect 100 percent cancer-free mice from the fields and imprison them in cages. They treat these innocent creatures like cooked excrement. They breed them with each other and feed them a "normal diet." After a few generations those mice are turned into what they call "pure inbred strains." According to them, those "inbred strains of mice" are in a special pathological condition, in which up to 80 percent of some strains are susceptible to "spontaneous" tumors of "unknown causes." This is a striking example of humanity's ignorance.

In reality, inbreeding is greatly beneficial if the offspring, which bear the recessive genetic weaknesses, are weeded out. Inbreeding purifies the strain and brings together the most potent elements of that creature's genetic history.

Each organism can only take so much cooked food. Every animal has hereditary weaknesses to certain diseases which make their appearance when the organism has reached its saturation point for cooked food. *Animals are only as strong as their weakest link.*

Researchers just close their eyes to the fact that the real physical, chemical, biological carcinogens are the very conditions that they have created for those poor mice. They have deprived them of their natural environment and food, isolated and enslaved them in metal cages. They are not allowed free exercise or sunlight. They live in air conditioned rooms, never breathing the open air.

It does not take an Annie Jump Cannon or a Nikola Tesla to discover the principles of disease and elucidate them to the world. All that any scientist has to do is free themselves from the mental and physical confines of the laboratory and direct her or his attention to the Sun, the moon, the oceans, the trees, and the flowers. They may then perceive Nature's precision and mentally plunge into the world's mysteries.

Can any scientist destroy the living Earth and construct a duplicate in its stead? That small sprouted lentil seed is an enormous world constructed by Nature itself. Scientists destroy that vivacious world and present humanity with their bread, amino acids, dead minerals, and salts. It would be interesting to know whether, after reading these lines, a scientist would still place their own knowledge above that of Nature.

What could be the cause of the spontaneous regression of tumors, if not some fortuitous change in the nutritional habits of the patient. There can be only one method for the successful treatment of cancer. The tumor must first be deprived of degenerated food.

It is not possible to confer on cancer cells the high qualities possessed by normal cells and to return them to the bosom of the community. Cancer cells must be starved.

Cancer starves on fruit. Fruits are rich in vitamins and other constituents of the highest nutritive value. Fruits are indeed magical. They perform tasks no artificial drug could ever match. All attempts to cure cancer by means of medicines and operations are absolutely futile and are doomed to utter failure. Prudent people never suffer from cancer if they do not upset the integrity of their raw food.

Cancer patients should immediately be placed on a light diet consisting exclusively of raw plant food, such as a honeydew melon or half a kilogram of grapes per day. This quantity is sufficient to keep the true body satiated, while the cancer cells, unable to find any cooked nourishment, gradually die. The cells could also be bathed in oxygen-rich fluids, such as wheatgrass juice. Cancer cells cannot exist in the presence of oxygen. Sunlight, fresh air, mild exercise, laughter, and loving/sexual relationships speed up the process. Let us give people a choice: eat raw or perish. Some people would rather die than take responsibility for their own life.

Cooked food is poison.

Chapter 13

Drug Therapy

"Nearly all people die of their medicines, and not of their illnesses."
— Moliere

All artificial drugs and medicines are symptomatic. They serve as numbing agents to give temporary relief to the patient or to conceal the symptoms of disease. In no way can they take the place of those raw nutrients which are unwittingly destroyed by cooking.

Drugs merely interfere with the purgative processes of the body, trapping even more poisons within the body which eventually cause far more damage to the organism in the end. Those who wish to maintain or regain their health must not pin their hopes on doctors, pharmacists, or other drug dealers; rather they must abstain from consuming unnatural foods and drugs, and must live according to the Laws of Nature — by eating raw.

This is the true, safe, and scientific way, whereas drug therapy is a mindcrime. It is an illusion, a self-deception, a veritable magic show with all the smoke and mirrors. Your philosopher, Friedrich Nietzsche, called drugs "the lashes of the whip."

The truth of what we are saying can be easily proven by the most basic scientific experiment: divide any group of ill patients into two groups; treat one group with drugs, medicines, and cooked foods and the other group with one hundred percent raw foods; then compare the two results. This is the most basic and decisive test imaginable; it refutes every argument against eating raw.

Below are just a *couple* of examples of the deplorable ignorance associated with drug therapy:

1. Pain is the body's warning cry, a sign that something is wrong. Doctors should focus on eliminating the source of the pain, but instead, choose to deaden the nerves that convey the sensation of this danger to the brain and confuse the body with a dose of poison. Meanwhile, the disease takes its inevitable course, aggravated now by the harmful effects of the drugs.

2. When the passages of the arteries grow narrow by being filled with impurities, the heart has to use greater force to circulate the blood through the body. As a result the blood pressure rises. Since no one wants to accept responsibility for their own health, the notion of cleaning out the arteries by fasting and eating raw foods is totally overlooked. Instead, people would rather get a prescription from their doctor for drugs that temporarily stimulate and widen the arteries. So long as the efficacy of the poison lasts, the blood flows through the vessels more freely and the blood pressure falls. However, as soon as its effect fades, the vessels return to their former constriction, all the more weakened by the action of the drugs used.

When a certain disease draws to itself the harmful currents of unnatural foods, the organism of the patient acquires a partial immunity from other diseases. For example, people who suffer from diabetes, atherosclerosis, and certain infectious diseases are less subject to cancer. Because of this, insane experiments have even been made to subject people to the influence of various bacteria for the alleged prevention of cancer. The same thing takes place on a smaller scale during vaccinations, when, by inducing milder forms of a disease children are "safeguarded" against serious attacks later on. The moment people decide to safeguard the health of their children by natural laws, such unnatural measures become exposed for their contradictory effects. Innocent children will be freed from state-mandated mutilations and the whole idea of vaccination will be tossed into the ashbin of history.

There has never been a vaccine, drug, or medicine created by humanity that did not have multiple, harmful side-effects.

Generally, drugs are held responsible for only those complications and reactions which immediately and violently kill the victim. Even then only one in a thousand of those complications is actually recorded; the rest are tossed into oblivion. Rarely, if ever, is a pharmaceutical company held accountable for the incredible crimes they commit.

All drugs are incredibly dangerous, from aspirin to AZT. You may not think that aspirin is dangerous. What would happen if someone consumed 50 aspirin pills? They would be poisoned. So, somehow, a small dose of poison is good? There is no such thing as moderation, only excess.

Medicines, synthetic vitamins, and organic extracts, by which people wish to replace the nutritive constituents of natural foods burned in the kitchen, may kill people at a lightning speed. Such artificial concoctions, especially these potent prescription medicines are not always eliminated by the body but are many times stored up for months, years, even decades. The body eventually becomes saturated and sensitive. People who wish to turn a blind eye to the responsibility of those drugs in causing more deaths and hideous diseases, tend to lay the blame on the "over-sensitiveness of the body." As to the cause of this over-sensitiveness, they somehow pass over this question entirely.

In the present age of mass communication it is ridiculous to observe how the most dangerous drugs are popularized by ad campaigns with songs, testimonials, and pictures suggesting more drug use. Throughout the entire Western world pharmacology has become a multi-trillion dollar industry engaged in ruthless commercialism and profiteering.

Raw-foodism will at once put an end to the use of all kinds of drugs and vaccines, because without illnesses the raison d'être for drug therapy disappears. The loathsome diseases of civilization are the consequence of the degeneration of natural foods; they can only be conquered by a return to a sane diet. All attempts to conquer diseases by means of drugs are extremely senseless and bizarre experiments which are doomed to failure. Their deplorable consequences are right out there in front of everyone's face, plain to see.

New types of diseases continually appear; slight illnesses give way to more serious disorders. As a result, people continually develop new kinds of vaccines and serums, discover stronger antibiotics, and gradually become involved in a labyrinth of errors, complications, and disasters which eventually spiral down into some dank, dark pit of despair.

Medical science, as we know it, must be abandoned for good. Its only positive aspect lies in its trauma repair and recovery techniques, but even they are severely flawed. All honest and well-spirited doctors and "health" professionals must at once rise up and take active steps to prevent the proliferation of more misinformation on the subject. The destruction of the integral raw materials designated for the human body must be prevented.

Cooked food is poison.

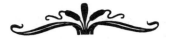

Chapter 14

Cooking = Extinction

"Drug paraphernalia such as stoves, toasters, coffee machines, refrigerators, and ovens are futile relics of a dead age. Anyone who continues to cling to them are like poisoned maggots clinging to a cooked-food corpse."
— **Nature's First Law**

Many species of animals have once inhabited this Earth and have then met with complete extinction owing to adverse environmental conditions. Today it is with their own hands that humans are creating such adverse conditions as will one day eliminate them from the face of the globe. The process of food degeneration creates an exact, paralleled increase in the variety and frequency of genetic mutations and various diseases. Before the passing of many more generations, people will die of cardiovascular diseases, cancer, or unnatural activities prior to reaching the age of puberty and will not have the opportunity to sexually reproduce. On the basis of the alarming speed at which those diseases have increased during the last few decades, it is easy to foresee that, should humans still persist in their folly, that fateful day may not be far off.

People who point out the benefits of cooked-eating and drug therapy are like businesspeople who, on the verge of bankruptcy, blame everyone but themselves and their own stale modes of thinking for their failure. The ultimate result of every business must be judged by its bottom line — no business can operate at a loss. *Nature judges by success, never by theory.*

Let us just look at what benefits and advantages the civilized masses have been able to acquire for themselves by their discoveries of cookery and medicine, in comparison with those enjoyed by countless other animals. Nothing, save the fact that although humans are one of the most perfect beings on this Earth, they are far more subject to various illnesses than any other creature.

After the discovery of vitamins humans should have had the common sense to perceive the way that cooking disintegrates those vitamins. They should have put an end to that waste once and for all and should have safeguarded natural foodstuffs from degeneration. But so great is the charm of cooked food that it thwarts all such attempts at reform. Remember, addiction conquers science. While still clinging fast to cooked food, humans try to penetrate into the secrets of nutrition and eugenics. It seems that biologists and laboratory technicians are trying to recognize those constituents that are destroyed in cooking and processing, and then replace them by synthetic substances. Is it not foolishness to burn and destroy those essential constituents by one's own hands, to become ill, to stand on the brink of the grave and then make hopeless attempts to save one's self by deceptive means? Is it not pure folly to actually believe that the strength of a race could be increased on cooked food?

Humans were once a higher, superior kind of being. What is left is only a remnant of the original, the result of cooking, subsequent degeneration, and bad breeding. However, by natural nutrition, one may still resurrect from extinction the true model of the species and experience a glimpse of what cannot be described.

By the research carried out on separate varieties of fruits, vegetables, and grains cooked-food-addicted biologists themselves prove that natural foodstuffs possess the properties which put a halt to every kind of degeneration. But people do not wish to admit that the human organism will remain free from those debilitations if it is fed exclusively on natural foodstuffs from childhood onwards. Right from the beginning, internal corruption created by cooked food has deprived most people of their ability to think clearly — and then science yields its place to addiction.

Addiction is synonymous with extinction.

Cooked food is poison.

Chapter 15

Raw-Foodism Produces Results

"Let food be your medicine and medicine be your food."
— Hippocrates

Progressive doctors condemn drug therapy. Some of them are so disappointed with the inefficacious results obtained from drug treatment that they abandon medical practice and devote themselves to the study of holistic science along with the fundamentals of prophylaxis — the prevention of disease. In this century, the most famous have been Bircher-Benner, the famous Swiss physician, and Max Gerson, the famous German physician.

At the onset of Bircher-Benner's medical career, he became so disillusioned with the current methods of therapeutics that upon discovering the nutritive values of natural foodstuffs, he began to cure his patients by the help of natural nutrition, without any drugs. Very soon a great number of patients, who had been unsuccessfully treated by various doctors all over the world, went to his sanitarium in Zurich. In a very short time they obtained a complete cure by means of a strictly raw-vegetarian diet.

Max Gerson cured himself of paralyzing migraines through an apple/raw-food diet. Later, he prescribed the diet to not only his headache suffering patients but to all his patients. He and his patients enjoyed "miraculous" results.

But Bircher-Benner and Max Gerson regarded raw food-stuffs as a "therapeutic means," not as the only diet fit for humanity. As if humans were obliged to nourish themselves on unnatural foodstuffs right from their childhood and then, having become ill, to be cured by the "therapeutic diet" in their advanced age! This apparent paradox had its definite reasons. First of all, there is nobody in the world, not even the foremost experts in raw nutrition, that realizes that cooked-eating is an addiction and that the desire people feel for cooked food is neither hunger nor the biological demand of the cells.

As physicians, Bircher-Benner and Gerson had been trained to address symptoms and to cure existing diseases. Nobody would have paid them any fees, or even taken him seriously, if they had publicly advocated a system of nutrition that would have kept humankind free from all diseases. Some doctors have been quoted as saying that if people ate like they were supposed to, they would lose four-fifths of their business. How much more obvious can it be?

Before a decision is made to undergo any surgery, the patient must give raw-foodism a chance. If the damaged organ has not completely lost its complement of active cells, it will regain its full working capacity. The diseased cells will be purged, healthy cells will grow in their stead. There is always immediate rejuvenation and a chance to get back under the sun and nighttime stars.

The final cure of every disease is entirely in the hands of patients themselves. The cause behind all the loathsome diseases of civilization is to be found in the kitchen fire. With the disappearance of that fire all the sufferings of the human race will also disappear. 100% raw-foodism not only acts as a preventative to every kind of illness, but it also clears the mind and heals the body of present diseases, provided that the affected organs still retain some signs of life.

To give just one example, we may look at cardio-vascular diseases. In some areas of North America and northern Europe, the mortality rate for heart disease is more than half the total mortality rate, and the ratio keeps on increasing. All the drugs which supposedly prevent such diseases are a total sham. By poisoning the body, irritating it, or by deadening the nerves and stimulating the heart muscle, they deprive the organism of its energy reserves. Take note of the fact that doctors are themselves the principal victims of heart-related diseases.

Yet among all diseases, cardio-vascular disorders are the most amenable to treatment. Raw-foodism puts an end to all those senseless deaths.

If heart patients should perchance take refuge in the Laws of Nature and change over to a raw diet, they would instantly feel an improvement in their condition. From the first moment of eating raw the blood vessels begin to cleanse. The heart and valves obtain a new lease on life with a fresh complement of active cells; they regain their proper elasticity and firmness. By eating raw foods, a once death-stricken heart patient may look forward to a healthy life of forty to fifty more years.

It is ridiculous to regard more than fifty percent of all deaths as "sudden" or "unexpected." When we see cheeseburgers and pizza entering the mouths of unsuspecting victims, we picture the degeneration that will soon be taking place in the walls of their heart and blood-vessels. We almost laugh at the unnatural behaviors that result from such feeding patterns. We have closed our hearts to pity for those who know of raw-foodism and choose to ignore it.

At the present moment there are two opposing views on nutrition. One of them defends raw-foodism, the other favors cooked-foodism; one of them advocates vegetarianism, the other prefers an animal diet or a combination (omnivorous) diet of cooked animals and plants. True science is not politics. The one who holds the wrong point of view has no right to impose erroneous and harmful opinions on innocent children. It is the absolute imperative demand of our times that these two view-points should be examined by international scientific and cultural circles, free from the sway of greed, delusion, and ignorance, so that the one that is wrong can be condemned, while the true one can be announced to the public and put into general practice. Our organization, Nature's First Law, is a vehicle for this process. We are taking forbidden information and placing it into the hands of those who can use it and know what to do with it.

Most simple-minded people do not wish to penetrate the depth of the problem. People believe that the idea of raw-food eating is not something that can be realized quickly and that sensible humans will not be ready to abandon their deep-rooted habits. But this is the voice of addiction, not of science. Science must be separated from addiction. Intelligent people must first admit that raw foodstuffs are the only real "medicines" suitable for the human organism; after which let those who wish to degenerate their own raw-food materials do so to their hearts' content.

We must make the use of the experience gained from raw-foodism to correct the false notions prevalent in the science of nutrition. This is truly an era of Orwellian "Newspeak" where the most essential foodstuffs are regarded as harmful, and the really harmful foodstuffs are recommended as wholesome. It must be clearly recognized that, without any exception, in all those cases where raw foodstuffs are forbidden to the weak, the sick, and the sufferers of stomach disorders and other ailments, it is precisely those forbidden foodstuffs that would heal, sustain, and strengthen the patients.

In such cases it is no longer a question of breaking off a bad habit. The situation is so bad, that in many hospitals patients who ask for fruit are denied. The patient feels sick of cooked food, but doctors and nurses persuade her or him to continue eating it so as to gain strength and weight. In other words, they hasten death by compelling the sick to eat those very foods that have been the cause of their illness and incapacity. The correction of misunderstandings of this kind alone will reduce the number of untimely deaths by fifty percent.

In order to convince everybody of the truth of these statements there is no other means but to put raw-foodism into practice for a few months. This experiment should be tried by every sensible person. It is in this way that a final end will be put to the existing erroneous and contradictory viewpoints on nutrition.

In the light of raw-foodism the basic principles of nutrition no longer remain confined to universities and research institutes; rather they become matters of primary importance to all humankind. The scientific names of thousands of foodstuffs, their complicated formulae, and the long, tiresome descriptions of their nutritive properties and supposed benefits can be summed up in just three words which are understandable to everyone: "Raw Plant Food" — the complete raw materials for the human machine.

Thus raw-foodism becomes an ideal apart from the science of medicine, an ideal that is explainable not by scientific formulae, but by logic; its proofs being the irrefutable Laws of Nature and the conclusive results obtained from basic experience.

Cooked food is poison.

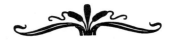

Chapter 16

Whole Food Is Best

*"Health is Beauty, and the most perfect
Health is the most perfect Beauty."*
— William Shemstone

The human body is one of the most perfect and at the same time one of the most complicated machines in the world. It may be appropriately regarded as a huge world of organic machines and systems in the sense that every cell, taken separately, is in itself a complicated machine which, in its own turn, consists of numerous other machines. Up to the present, research scientists have been able to discover as many as ten-thousand parts in each cell. Every gland or organ is composed of billions of such cells, and it is from the combination of those glands, organs, blood, bones, and skin that the human body is formed.

In order that they may carry out their functions properly, these highly complicated machines and systems must be provided with raw materials. Each type of raw plant food contains millions of different substances, each of which has its special duty to perform in the general organization of the human organism. All those substances are constructed by the help of sunlight and are concentrated in plant bodies. For instance, a sunflower seed, a chard leaf, or a jalapeño pepper contains all those nutritive constituents that are essential to an animal organism. Although those constituents differ in various plants as regards their composition and arrangement, this matters little. After their introduction into the organism these materials are broken down and synthesized again. During this process one substance is changed into another substance. Thus, the organism is able to change the quantities of the various constituents according to its needs, but in the absence of a certain chemical element it can not bring that missing element into being inside the organism or substitute it by another element.

For instance, it has not been possible to discover in the laboratory any massive concentrations of calcium, vitamins, or proteins in clover, yet it is from clover and from still more common grasses that animals take all their vitamins and mineral salts, and construct their massive bones, flesh, muscle, and fat. In other words, in place of the milk, butter, cheese, liver, and dead animal muscle that short-sighted people recommend as sources of calcium, phosphorus, vitamins, and "fully balanced" proteins, clover alone may be recommended, for it is from clover that all those substances originate. Therefore, it is completely meaningless, worthless, and even harmful to claim that such-and-such a foodstuff is rich in a certain vitamin, while another abounds in a particular mineral, because, apart from misleading and confusing people, such claims do not serve any purpose.

The main functions of nutritive constituents in the organism are threefold. First of all they serve as building material for the construction and renewal of cells, then they produce the necessary energy for putting those cells into motion and giving warmth to the body, and lastly they supply the specialized cells with the raw materials needed for their productive activities.

It is imperative that you should look after your organism with the same care as engineers look after their machines. Accordingly, for the operation of the foregoing threefold functions you must supply your body with all the necessary nutritive constituents as an integral whole and in the same balanced proportions as Nature presents them. Otherwise, should there be a deficiency in any of the constituents, this fact will inevitably have an adverse effect on the construction and working of the organism.

But how do the "civilized" humans of today treat their own bodies? They dissipate, burn, kill, and upset the integrity of raw-food materials and then they fill their stomachs at random with the dead and poisonous corpses containing only a few thousand denatured substances. In this way their consumption of certain food constituents may exceed the normal requirements of their organism by hundreds of times, with a corresponding deficiency in the intake of some other constituent.

The most "learned" nutrition experts usually consider bacterial contamination, moldy putrefaction, and fermentation to be the only defects of foodstuffs. They view as nutritious, wholesome, and normal all those foods that are sealed, clean, and well-cooked. They do not seem the least bit worried about the deplorable absence of essential living vitamins and minerals. When they are reminded of this fact, they senselessly reply that they eat fruit too, but never even fathom that fruit is all they should be eating.

It is necessary to emphasize the fact that cooking is not the only factor that causes a loss in the nutritive value of foodstuffs. Dead and denatured foods such as pickles, unsprouted nuts, and essene bread also are problematic for the digestive organs. Dried straw is not a perfect food for grazing animals, in spite of the fact that it is able to keep them alive. A perfect foodstuff could be the stalk of wheat if it is eaten green in the spring and also sprouted wheatberries in the winter. For caged animals such as parrots and parakeets, one type of plant food cannot be regarded as total nutrition. Those animals have gone through their evolution in free Nature, feeding simultaneously on grasses, leaves, fruits, and vegetables. That is why particular cases of diseases occur among those animals that have been denied, through the intervention of humans, the foodstuffs proper to the requirements of their cells. Nevertheless, at no time are the organs of animals feeding on the untampered, dried plant foods subject to such perils as human organs are; nor are microbes of such terror to them as they are to humans, for the simple reason that they have no kitchen.

The cells that are produced from fish, pasta, baked squash, soy milk, cornbread, yogurt, beer, etc. are devoid of the capacity to perform any useful work. The active, specialized, and completely healthy cells of the human body are born exclusively of raw fruits and vegetables. Incredibly, those foods maintained in their natural and living state are looked upon by the cooked-food addict as some sort of dessert.

Everybody should now be able to realize the enormity of the crime committed by parents who tell their children not to spoil their "appetite" with fruit before dinner because they must eat all their cooked food. This is tantamount to telling them not to eat the millions of different raw-food materials that are essential for their organism and to instead wait for the dead and lifeless corpses of a few animals which they will soon receive in the form of a meal.

Cooked-eaters are happy at the thought of counting calories. A calorie has nothing to do with the way the human body processes food. When the number of active muscular cells is small (and even those are weak, diseased, and devoid of elasticity), the greater part of the calories remain unused. After causing a considerable amount of trouble to the body, these caloric foods leave the organism in the form of unwanted heat, and are lost to no avail. When you light a fire in the open air, the energy of that fire is uselessly lost, but when you burn that fire in the motor of a machine, it fully serves its purpose. The body temperature of a cooked-food human is 37 degrees Celsius (98.6 degrees Fahrenheit), the body temperature of a raw-food human is 36 degrees Celsius (96.8 degrees Fahrenheit). By means of cooked foods addicts introduce into their bodies an intake of calories three to four times in excess of the functional requirements of their organism. The calories that are obtained from raw food-stuffs fully serve their purpose, because such foodstuffs are accompanied with all the factors necessary for the utilization of those calories.

The absurd process of counting calories must be abandoned for good. Most people do not even know what a calorie is. A calorie is the amount of heat energy required to raise the temperature of one gram of water one degree Celsius. This really has nothing to do with nutrition. A vast amount of literature has been concocted dealing with the study of the separate constituents in foodstuffs; a study which is no longer confined to scientific circles, but has become highly popularized and even mandated on cooked-food packages. Yet, the great attention paid to individual constituents springs from the fact that their integrity has been upset and as a result the body has been deprived of an important part of them. The study of individual nutritive constituents is still in its most elementary stage and not one in a thousand of its secrets is known to humanity. Hence, that study should at present be confined to scientific circles and all pointless experiments for the testing of individual nutrients, especially of animal proteins, synthetic vitamins and minerals, should be carried out on ignorant, unwilling subjects, such as violent prisoners, and never on innocent people or animals. In humanity's present imperfect state of knowledge it is most dangerous to experiment on the human body. In any case, there is no need to have recourse to artificially-made individual constituents, when we have them all at our constant disposal in their wonderful integrity, and especially since no nutritive substance can serve any useful purpose if it is taken in isolation.

Biologists and doctors have a duty to encourage people to avoid the separation of nutritive constituents. These elements must be consumed together, in their naturally balanced proportions, as they exist in the living cells. How preposterous it is to talk about the usefulness of individual nutritive constituents, when these elements are actually indispensable. And how ridiculous it is to speak of the benefits of any particular vitamin (as pseudo-nutritionists typically do) when each functions as part of the vital whole.

Cooked food is poison.

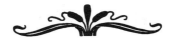

Chapter 17

The Origin Of Disease

"It is my experience that aside from a few human affections, the only thing that gives lasting and untainted pleasure in the world, is the pursuit of truth and the destruction of error."
— **Thomas H. Huxley**

In the course of millions of years, some primitive unicellular organisms underwent a long evolutionary process facilitated by the ever increasing quality of nutritive substances created as byproducts of advancing organic life. During that evolutionary development, those cells perfected themselves and gave birth to ever more complex organisms, including human beings. We can see a brief synopsis of this biological development in the embryo of an animal, from the instant of fertilization to its full development. The same process is repeated during the development of individual human cells.

Let us take a gland that is composed of a billion cells. These cells are of numerous kinds, each of which has its particular function or duty to perform. There are muscle cells, epithelial cells, nerve cells, and host of other cell types. The main function of these gland cells is the secretion of fluids.

The glands of a cooked-foodist contain a full complement of cells, but only twenty to twenty-five percent of those cells are fit for any useful work. Protein alone, especially the dead, cooked, animal protein which is regarded by short-sighted people as the perfect building material, can (at most) call into existence only the simplest, most primitive cell structures. In their arrangement these cells resemble those primitive organisms which first made their appearance on this planet in the earliest stages of evolutionary development. These cells are constructed with improper building materials: imperfect proteins, cooked fats, and dehydrated carbohydrates.

In a given gland, every specialized cell possesses particular mechanisms which can only acquire the capacity for active work and organization by the supply of special nutritive constituents. The raw materials necessary for the productive functions of those mechanisms can be provided solely by highly-evolved, raw nutrients. No bee can create honey from the nectar of a cooked flower.

When the special constituents do not reach the cell in sufficient quantities, its development is thereby slowed and/or stunted. This gives rise to a variety of atavistic and diseased cells, such as fatty, anaplastic, malignant, or cancer cells, macrophages, megakaryocytes, polykaryocytes, etc.

Within the gland, not only do most of the cells not attain specialization, but also the raw materials (necessary for the secretion of fluids) do not reach the few cells that still retain the ability to do work. As an inevitable result, the gland is not able to maintain its proper level of production. It has become diseased. Improper development and crude functioning of the cells may also occur in all the other organs and systems, resulting in the appearance of corresponding diseases.

Sometimes a certain gland or organ is so damaged that its removal is recommended by a cooked-food surgeon. Instead of adopting a raw-food regimen, people go through an incredible hassle, discomfort, and expense to remove the gland or organ and then pride themselves on the performance of such a "miracle." To a raw-foodist it is quite clear that no drugs or surgeries can restore a degenerated gland or organ to its normal condition and return it to its proper capacity for work.

When due account is taken to Nature's First Law the cause of no disease remains hidden; everything becomes as clear as a summer day. As soon as the number of normal, active cells decreases through a decrease in the quantity of natural foods consumed, the organs fail in their operations. Their yield becomes poor, insufficient and defective. As a result the given organs become ill and protection from the elements becomes minimal. Again, because comparatively few active cells remain, the walls of the heart distend and the valves become damaged. The sensitive linings of the mucous membranes, skin, intestines, and stomach become irritated and erode, creating allergies. The capillaries dilate, then burst. The teeth decay; the hair turns gray and falls out. The joints become suppositories for cooked nightshade plant extracts and uric acid — they eventually wear out. The walls of the blood vessels become layered in cooked animal deposits. Stones form in the liver and bladder. Every type of disease makes its appearance. It is quite easy to explain the causes of all this madness: cooked food.

The nutritive value of foodstuffs is found, not in a variety of foods constituting the "four food groups" or some "balanced pyramid of nutrition," but in a variety of elements composing those foodstuffs. The commonest grass is richer in the quantity of its nutritive elements than an entire buffet of cooked food. This is the verdict of science.

Every year, all over the world, countless medical conferences take place for the prevention of diseases. Categorically, after discoursing for hours about unimportant, secondary subjects, the foremost representatives of medical science gather around richly decorated tables for a full-course meal of cooked food. They ignore basic, fully-balanced foods, which are formed perfectly in Nature's own laboratory and proceed to stuff their faces with four or five types of cooked animals and dead vegetables. Worse still, many of them complete their regimen of nutrition with alcoholic beverages, ice cream, coffee, and cigarettes. Anyone with even the least bit of common sense must surely agree that this is a ridiculous form of nutrition. It is high time people seriously consider making a fundamental change in their present feeding customs.

During the vietnam war, some American prisoners of war were condemned to death by being fed a diet consisting exclusively of cooked meat. Many did not survive longer than one month, whereas, in the event of complete fasting a person may survive as long as one hundred days. This clearly demonstrates that not only is cooked meat a degenerate foodstuff, but with the toxins that it produces, it is really a poison that kills the victim fairly quickly.

It is a widely stated proverb that "three billion people cannot be wrong." They are when they consume cooked rice.

Prolonged consumption of cooked rice causes stunted growth. Additionally, it is a known fact that people who consume vast amounts of polished rice, such as those people living in eastern and southern Asia, are subject to beriberi — a deficiency disease of the peripheral nervous system characterized by partial paralysis of the extremities, emaciation, and anemia. This disease is not caused by thiamine deficiency as is generally supposed; such a deficiency is only a symptom of polished rice addiction.

White bread and all the ancillary products created from white flour have characteristics similar to those of polished rice. The same is true of refined sugar and clarified fats. It is amusing when people have long arguments over which is healthier: butter or margarine. That is like asking what would feel better: a gunshot or a deep stab wound?

Credulous people naively believe that whatever the stomach readily accepts cannot be harmful, whereas white rice, white flour, and white sugar, which are the most harmful of all foods, induce no immediate reaction in the cooked-foodist's stomach.

It is these foodstuffs that comprise the staple diet of the cooked-food eater and are the main factors that eventually cause premature death. They kill under the guise of infectious diseases, anemia, cancer, diabetes, mental illness, diarrhea, etc. Sometimes they kill at the age of only one year, at other times at the age of six, twenty, sixty, or eighty years, depending on the relative proportions one consumes of the two categories of food (raw versus cooked), each person's inherited genetic potential, and how much food is consumed — typically the less a person eats, the longer that person lives (that is why there is no such thing as an obese centenarian).

Indeed, the subject of quantities of food consumed begs further attention. It is a scientific fact that systematic under-feeding has been the most effective method discovered for extending the life of not only warm-blooded mammals, but also of fish and worms.

We appeal to the common sense of all people including doctors and "health-care" professionals. They must seriously consider this matter. Our statements are not mere hypotheses, but irrefutable facts demonstrable not only by the most elementary Laws of Nature, but also by the final and positive results experienced by ourselves and other raw-foodists throughout the world.

Hospitals should be replaced by greenhouses where people can relax, receive massages, live and breathe the luxuriant air of green plant life, and eat fruit.

The best means of preventing and curing human illnesses, and at the same time raising the standards of living for all intelligent people, is for every media and communications establishment to make this book available to the masses.

Most people are not sensible. It is impossible to make everybody a raw-foodist. The mass mind is atrophied from little use. People have been taught what to think, not how to think.

It is, however, essential that people be acquainted with proper nutritional information from the earliest age so that they may free themselves from unnatural propensities and vices. People certainly need to know that it is not chicken soup, bread, brown rice, eggs, dead (pasteurized) orange juice, but the living grape, lime, cucumber, carrot, and wheatgrass, that gives both them and their children health and vitality. In our own cases, we can testify that our strength is so enhanced that we typically spend only four to six hours sleeping and engage in more activities by ten in the morning than most people do in an entire day.

Once intelligent people are acquainted with the harms caused by cooked foods, they will naturally try to avoid them. There will arise a great number of sensible people who, drowning in the voice of their own addictions, will follow our example and by the practice of complete raw-eating will assure the perfect health of themselves and their families. People who have lost all hope due to threats of terminal illness or have become disfigured by unnatural obesity will realize that, by strict obedience to Natural Law, they (within a few months) will be able to attain the health that has always eluded them.

Some people wonder what connection nutrition could have with the functioning of the eyes, the nerves, the skin, as though any part of the body could carry on its operations without raw materials. What substances might one possibly find in a meatball sandwich doused in tomato sauce and cheese that could give light to the eyes, organize the wonderful operations of the nerves, or moisten and soothe the skin? People advance all sorts of hypothetical conjectures to explain the causes of nervous diseases, but they do not pay the least bit of attention to the most essential factor — the quality of the materials supplied to the nerves.

The dietary regime of the cooked-food addict is full of fatal contradictions. Harmful foodstuffs are recommended as useful, while essential foodstuffs are represented as harmful and strictly forbidden. This is because the experience of the cooked-food addict is based on the immediate, apparent, and contradictory effects of foods and on erroneous calculations made within the laboratory. Untold masses of unknowing people perish as a result of those contradictory and erroneous calculations.

The most reliable guide is the fundamental and perfect experience of the raw-foodist. Raw-foodism exposes all the errors, contradictions, and misunderstandings that exist in medical science and popular media mythology. It is necessary to exponentially multiply the concept of raw-foodism throughout the world.

Cooked food is poison.

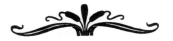

Chapter 18

Children

*"If you must hold yourself up to
your children as an object lesson...
hold yourself up as an example and not as a warning."*
— **Bernard Shaw**

"Those having torches will pass them on to others."
— **Plato**

The gravest terrorism is the terrorism inflicted upon children when they are forced to copy the cooked-food addictions of their parents. What right do parents have to pass along their own addictions to an infant? By what right do parents introduce foods burned, destroyed, and killed by heat and flame into the organism of an innocent newborn child? Is this not the most ruthless of all crimes? Is it not in effect a homicide, a brutal filicide?

In reality, all cooked-food parents are filicides. Nobody dies a natural death. All deaths are the result of diseases, degenerations, and unnatural behaviors caused by eating cooked, dead, and denatured beverages and foods. Cooked parents must fully realize that the responsibility of every one of their childrens' illnesses and disorders rests squarely upon their shoulders. The body of every adult — both female and male — who desires a child, must be completely cleansed of toxins. This is the only way to extinguish any threat of genetic damage or impaired health in the child. Cooked adults must seriously weigh this matter before persisting in their usual mistaken course.

During the first few years of life, the infant carries on a terrible struggle against unnatural nutrition. This is plainly evident from the numerous ailments (e.g., throat infections, stomach disorders, earaches, etc.) with which they are afflicted and from the alarmingly high rate of infant mortality. All of these are evidence of the organism's struggle to "adapt" to cooked, dead, and denatured foods. Babies are newly-constructed, perfect organic machines. They would never become ill if they were supplied with the natural foods for which they were designed.

When, after three or four months of forced cooked-eating, the organs of an infant child begin to operate irregularly, ignorant doctors step in to prescribe two or three types of synthetic vitamins (as if they could ever replace the synergetic properties contained in the tens of thousands of compounds destroyed over the kitchen fire) or, even worse, to prescribe medicines which create all sorts of dysfunctions.

After lying in the alimentary canal for days, masses of meat, cheese, and eggs undergo putrefaction and cause inflammation of the intestines. The most common symptom of this condition is diarrhea. When a child shows signs of diarrhea, myopic, cooked-food parents place the blame on a few fruit-skins observable in the feces. Nobody asks how it is possible that fruit-skins can cause any inflammation in the bowels of the child when, without undergoing any putrefaction or decay, they typically leave the body unchanged in less than a day. The whole tragedy arises from the fact that people regard meat, cheese, and eggs as normal, while fruit is something secondary, a "dessert" or "snack" which may or may not be eaten. Sometimes it is even considered necessary to forbid a child to eat fruit so as "not to upset the stomach." Certain religions even go so far as to instill this nonsense with a story about "the forbidden fruit."

The foundation of every heart-attack and cancer is laid with the first morsel of cooked food given to a baby, even when the final form of the disease makes its appearance at a most advanced age.

Little children never cry without reason. They should never experience a restless night, suffer from stomach disorders, ear infections, or even fevers. All these are the result of cooked food and inorganic beverages such as: hot dogs, "baloney" sandwiches, potato chips, dried breakfast cereal, soda, and pasteurized cow's milk.

All this absurdity would end instantaneously if the home fire was extinguished forever. That is where we step in; we fight kitchen fires and save lives.

Health begins with breast feeding. Breast feeding is the absolute command of Nature. Mothers need to unlearn modesty and men need to unlearn jealousy, because nursing should be in the great outdoors under a tree not in some dark, secluded room (artificial cave).

As a result of unnatural nutrition many mothers have no milk to nurse their babies, and so they resort to inorganic baby formulas and jarred moldy peaches. Quite naturally, the child becomes pudgy, pale, inwardly emaciated, and a screaming mess.

Such children can be restored to health within two weeks simply by being fed a couple tumblers of freshly made fruit juice each day. But cooked-food dietitians and doctors ignore the necessity of fruit and instead carry out the most abominable experiments on the degenerated body of the child. They draw the child's anemic blood and then try to nourish the child with dried milk, meat extracts, artificial vitamins, and various drugs. Disregarding the harmonious balance of the nutritional elements generously provided by Nature, they experiment on the emaciated body of the child by means of a few vitamins and minerals about which they have obtained some fragmentary information in their laboratories. If that child does not obtain natural foodstuffs, love, fresh air, and sunlight upon the skin, s/he dies; and such deaths occur daily in the thousands. But, what is still more terrible, many naive dietitians and doctors prevent such children from eating raw fruit in the belief that their weak stomachs will not be able to digest it. Take heed of the fact that hospitals supply meat, bread, soup, milk, jello, coffee, ice cream, refined sugar, tea, white rice, artificial vitamins, and noisome medicines in great abundance, but rarely will you find a juice extractor or fresh pieces of fruit. Not only children, but people of all ages die in these hospitals. Nobody wishes to hold the unnatural system of nutrition responsible for those deaths.

Many adults argue that it is very difficult to completely abstain from cooked food. Very well, let them persist in their pernicious habits to their addiction's content. But what is it that compels these people to deprive young children and infants of essential raw nourishment?

In this age of "scientific advance," we still see numerous pallid, sickly children whose mothers resort to every kind of encouragement and threat to get those kids to eat chicken soup, dead orange juice, inorganic vitamins, jello, and ginger ale. Those same mothers strictly forbid them oranges and apples for being "indigestible," grapes and cherries for "causing diarrhea," and berries and melons for "giving rise to fever." How can we tolerate with indifference this deplorable state of affairs? Should we laugh or should we cry? Perhaps the methods by which addictions are passed from adults to their offspring is Nature's way of ending entire genetic lines.

There is certainly no Law of Nature which prevents parents from feeding their child fruit instead of candy, fresh juices instead of pasteurized cow's milk, bananas instead of meat and cheese. By eating raw foods children enjoy healthy, happy, long lives, whereas cooked foods lead them towards behavior which is inimical to the natural order. It is impossible for a child who is filled with cooked, dead, and poisonous extracts of food to behave naturally. Children desire raw foods with all their instinctive being. Nature ordains their indisputable right to these whole, living foods. Any parent or pediatrician with the least bit of common sense must act upon this information and prescribe a lifestyle for children accordingly.

The children in our families never have to ask for any fruits or vegetables. They are always seasonal varieties presented in plain sight, within reach, and in abundance.

In the name of every helpless child we appeal to all parents, scientists, scholars, anthropologists, and anybody involved in any governing body or authoritative position to put an immediate end to this terrible crime. Every day's delay costs thousands upon thousands of lives. Adults are free to commit suicide by sacrificing their lives to the absurd pleasures of cooked foods, but who has given them the right to massacre innocent children, especially as those foods, far from giving them any pleasure, merely fill those children with negative and violent emotions?

Children are smarter than cooked adults. Children are instinctively repelled by cooked food; they still have a strong alimentary instinct. They naturally desire colorful fruits and vegetables; they especially have an affinity for the soft fruits, such as bananas, grapes, kiwis, and berries.

Though peer pressure is strong, it is pure pessimism to argue that a raw-raised child will see others eating cooked abominations and thus desire those things. Instinct is strong if it is allowed to grow. But remember, by the law of imitation, adults become the role-models for their children. *Therefore, those who persist in their cooked habits while trying to raise their children naturally always run into difficulty.*

The first time these children try to eat cooked foods their bodies will throw it right out, an experience similar to that many people remember from the first time they ever tried alcohol or smoked cigarettes. There are millions of people who, after some experimentation, see the alcoholism and drug addiction of others and manage to stay away from it. Which heroin addict teaches her or his child to acquire that drug habit right from the cradle? What kind of sense prompts an adult to sacrifice their own offspring by getting them addicted to their loathsome habits in order to sanction and perpetuate their own addictions? Let parents first bring up their healthy children according to the Laws of Nature and then, after they grow up, let them leave their future course of action to their own free will, just as they do in the case of all other vices.

When it becomes apparent that cooked-eating is an unnatural habit, that it is the cause of all human illnesses, and that it is such a terrible addiction that once human beings fall prey to its remorseless grip they are seldom able to free themselves from its clutches, no parent will be able to remain indifferent. After learning of the truth, no loving parent can find justification in the contradictory advice of supposed authorities. Should parents persist in ignoring the voice of truth, they must take on the responsibility for ruining their child's health and undermining her or his future.

Everything is so simple; it is so obvious. Give your children fruit and you feed them for a day. Teach your children how to grow a garden and you feed them for a lifetime.

A person must be devoid of the most elementary judgment to replace millions of substances by a hundred substances, living cells by dead cells, fully-balanced raw materials by degenerated materials, natural nutriments by unnatural nutriments, sprouted wheat by bread, green peas by cooked meat, fresh fruit by jam.

On what scientific grounds are the food choices made for children forced into public education systems? The hamburgers, corn dogs, french fries, chocolate milk, brownies, candy, and soda should be immediately replaced by baskets of fresh, seasonal fruits and vegetables. Children should be able to eat from these baskets at all times of the day and in any quantity they prefer. Then it will be clear for everyone to see how, by the Laws of Nature, children will automatically begin to consume more fruits and vegetables and less degenerated food, thus assuring their own health and well-being.

Today's society is one in which parents are too apt to let their children run the show. You hear, "Well, my children won't eat vegetables" or, "My children don't like fruit." So, of course, in order to avoid a confrontation with their children, the parent gives them exactly what they want and then watch them abominate their bodies with a dinner of burgers and fries or macaroni and cheese. Then parents wonder why their child screams, cries, and is always ill. If only these parents would have the same authority in their childrens' diets as they do when the situation is a teachers' strike at school. These parents become violent and storm City Hall when their children are out of school (indoctrination center) for even one day. Today's youth has been weaned on the decadent nipple of television and a culture that feeds them lies. Raw-foodism will take them into the Truth.

Cooked food is poison.

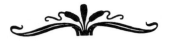

Chapter 19

Nature And The Vicious Cycle

"If you believe absurdities, you shall commit atrocities."
— Voltaire

We hereby publicly appeal to all scientists that they must confirm our views and declare to the entire world that cooked food is poison or, in the alternative, that they must prove that when natural foodstuffs are treated by heat and flame no losses are incurred in their nutritive elements or energy contents, no deaths of the living plant cells occur, and no changes take place in the constitution of the organic molecules. If they claim nothing is wrong with cooked food, they must further prove that Nature has made a mistake in not presenting us foodstuffs in their cooked state, that the operations carried out in laboratories, food processing plants, and kitchens are scientific measures aimed at correcting Nature's errors, and that synthetic vitamins have greater nutritional value than the vitamins found in Nature. Failing that, they must admit humanity's tragic mistake and do away with cooked meals once and for all. They must take refuge in the all-encompassing wisdom of Nature — this begins by ending the degeneration of foodstuffs. No natural creature ever tampers with its food. Let those who think that humans are meat-eaters consume their meat in its raw, freshly-killed state as every other carnivore does. Otherwise, they would be best off by shutting their mouths.

By what incredible arrogance do humans believe that they can upset the integrity of the raw materials created by Nature when, with all the "advances" of science, no one could possibly replicate, artificially, even the most basic single-celled organism. Even with the help of all the "newly-discovered" nutritive elements, scientists still are unable to feed an organism artificially without it falling into disarray. A great deal of hapless research has been conducted and considerable progress has been made in the recognition of various nutrients, but this information is meaningless, for every raw fruit and vegetable is a complete and whole food not devoid or lacking even when grown in weak soil and under harsh conditions.

Many people are quick to declare that plant foods must be "supplemented" with artificial vitamins and minerals due to the demineralization of the soil and the insane process of pesticide treatment. The "urgency" of nutrient depletion is a myth perpetuated by the synthetic-vitamin industry. If the plant still has enough energy and nutrition to put forth fruits and vegetables, then those foods are complete — their requisite nutrient base may be decreased, but their nutrient ratios are still perfect and they are still whole synergistic energy systems. When you eat a raw fruit or vegetable you consume every vitamin and trace mineral that exists. On an additional point, supplementing the diet with freshly made vegetable juice to get a full array of vitamins may benefit a cooked-foodist, but a raw-foodist will find it unnecessary.

Nutrient depletion itself is caused by cooked-food addiction. Most agricultural resources are sown, reaped, and then shipped off to various places to be fed to livestock or to be cooked in food-processing factories. 90% of the corn and soy beans in the U.S. are used to feed livestock. Livestock are ritualistically enslaved and slaughtered for their milk and flesh. All the massive resources put into those animals are then burned on the fire. If people cut out animal products from their diet soil depletion ends, not to mention all the water that will not be wasted. Twenty vegetarians can live off the land of one meat-eater. The vicious cycle of meat addiction in this mechanized world really defies description. Let no mistake be made about it, humanity's food choices are what is destroying the planet.

Obviously the ultimate goal is to eat homegrown fruits, vegetables, and herbs. Gardening is the purest of human pleasures. In the alternative one should seek out pesticide-free foods.

The best course of study is to delve into deep ecology through a careful analysis of the laws of natural plant and animal evolution and then to assist the work of Nature by using natural means to speed up that evolution. Under no circumstances should anybody undo the work of Nature and then try to falsify it under erroneous pretexts and misconceptions. This holds true for all aspects of human existence.

When someone fries a piece of eggplant or potato in oil, the process of destruction begins. It immediately begins to sizzle, shrivel, dehydrate, and carbonize; if the process continues, it eventually turns to ashes. That false, appetizing smell which tantalizes the addicted nostrils during the cooking process, is the last cry of those most valuable natural elements as they evaporate into thin air.

The terms "cooking," "grilling," "baking," and "microwaving" must never be given the connotation of preparing, constructing, or improving; rather they must be employed to convey a sense of death, pain, fire, and destruction. It is through those operations that people wantonly destroy the most valuable food substances and thus commit the most heinous crimes against Nature.

Cooked food is poison.

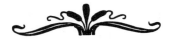

Chapter 20

The Eternal Law

"The law immutable, indestructible, eternal; not like those of today and yesterday, but made ere time began."
— **Sophocles**

As paradoxical as it may seem, Homo sapien, the most destructive animal of all time, is a fruitarian creature. It is humanity's cooked-food addiction which has divorced humanity from a natural state of living and unleashed a self-destructive terror upon this Earth. Cooked food is the bane of all existence.

Ignorant people actually think it is cruel to deprive children of the "pleasures" of cooked food. Such people must realize that cooked foods are not tasty at all; they seem tasty only to the cooked-food addict, just as cocaine seems tasty to the cocaine addict. Until now, there has been nobody on the planet to inform people of this simple truth, because from time immemorial people have been addicted to cooked food.

The organs of all creatures, from the earthworm to the moth, from the infant human baby to the cooked, denatured adult, are designed to process raw materials. You don't become a raw-foodist, you already are one — it is not some diet you do, it is something you are.

But at some point, usually early in life, you become a cooked-foodist, and that is the tragedy. Newborn children tremendously enjoy the tastes and satisfactions derived from fruits and their juices. They taste fantastic to the child, but are only a snack or dessert for the cooked adult. Children do not derive any pleasure whatsoever from the taste of cooked foods. They loathe and shun them with all their might; it is with great pain that they swallow those unwholesome materials. Children don't want to eat their vegetables because they are cooked! *But many parents cannot understand this; they are guided solely by unnatural traditions and severe addictions.* In their cooked minds they stress themselves out over keeping their children "well-fed" and thus continue to force those vile foods down their innocent childrens' throats. Such children end up totally addicted and their birthright of health and happiness corrupted.

Cooking is an unnatural activity. It is a lie which keeps being perpetuated at the family hearth generation after generation, millennia after millennia. It is well understood by some intelligent types that the key factor in getting a lie to be believed is the size of the lie. The broad masses of people, in the primitive simplicity of their minds, fall victim more easily to a big lie than a small one. And cooking is the most massive of all lies. A lie cannot be sustained in Nature. When you falsify Nature, you murder part of the world. Sooner or later, Nature smashes all lies. That is why Nature's First Law has arrived.

One day this world will once again be entirely raw-eaters — with or without human beings.

The universal adoption of raw-food eating is the only way to free humanity from those loathsome diseases of civilization. The propagation of raw-foodism must begin with newborn children, "terminally" ill people, great minds endowed with an extraordinary common sense and will-power, and sensible people all over the globe who can set an example for their families. The period of voluntary abstention from cooked food will last until the day when humanity is at last returned to a natural form of government and the governing authority resolves to declare raw-food eating mandatory, thus forcing the eternal Laws of Nature upon the ignorant, bumbling masses. In some future time the degeneration of essential raw materials necessary for the human organism will be declared an atrocious crime and will be punished by the severest penalties.

The supposed difficulty of abolishing cooked-food habits is no excuse for denying the harm done by them. It is essential for scientists to declare to the public that the operation of cooking, refining, and degenerating foodstuffs is unhealthy, unnatural, and dangerous, and that it is the source of all disease without any exception. The secondary question of putting raw-foodism into actual practice may then be left to the subsequent course of events.

Cooked-food experimentation has successfully degenerated into food addiction, diseases, medical science, and pharmacology. The ultimate purpose of medical science is to mend and restore mangled organs and psychological impairments, not profiteering and experimentation. In the place of medical science, raw-foodists have real science and health, the aim of which is to prevent all degenerations and to ensure a healthy, happy, long, and successful life for present and future generations. All human problems are caused by a violation of the Laws of Nature. Eating raw compels people to respect and nurture those laws.

Cooked food is poison.

Chapter 21

Anthropology

*"People who are ignorant of their evolutionary past
will defile their present and destroy their future."*
— **Nature's First Law**

When life first appeared on Earth, Nature had at its disposal only the most elementary building materials (carbon dioxide, water, oxygen, amino acids) from which it succeeded in creating the first single-celled organisms. Slowly, and in enigmatic epochs, over millions and millions of years of evolution the struggle for survival led to slightly more complicated structures building upon some of those already existing organisms. This arduous task has kept Nature busy for 4.5 billion years, during which time, single-celled plants have developed into fruit trees and, in subsequent conjunction, single-celled animals have developed into human beings.

All the living organisms in the world have descended from the same ancestors. During the course of time they have taken different evolutionary directions.

The physiological and genetic differences between Homo sapien and other highly-developed mammals are fundamentally very small. Just like Homo sapien, other highly-developed mammals have hearts, lungs, kidneys, wombs, livers, blood, bones, flesh, etc. Their organs demand exclusively raw materials, just as human organs do.

For all time mammals have sustained themselves exclusively on raw food. We must take note of the fact that when a zebra or giraffe consumes a leaf from a tree, it satisfies all the needs of its organism. In that single leaf, Nature has concentrated all those substances which are necessary to construct, differentiate, nourish, and energize new cells in the body of that animal. The plant organ or leaf comprises the fully-balanced raw materials destined by the far-sighted life-principle for that animal organism.

The most important difference in natural evolution between humans and other animals lies in the descent of the larynx, which allows breath control, and the development of the vocal chords, which allows speech and communication. Speech, communication, and the written word have allowed people to transmit complex thoughts from their own mind to the minds of others and thus to spread knowledge.

The history of proto-humanity is profoundly mysterious. What is known about the past is so infinitesimally small, that essentially almost nothing is known at all. Only 1,000 pieces have been found of a puzzle containing six million pieces. The anthropological theories that flood the media are nothing more than fantastic assumptions and conjectures put together by nescient researchers.

Simple probability indicates that the fossil records can only be test samples of life as it once existed on Earth. If evolution was truly a mechanical process of increasing fitness and utility as it has been taught, each sample should occasionally proffer up transitional types that are not particularly of one genus or another. Instead we find perfectly stable and unaltered forms persevering through eons. They seem to appear suddenly and always in their definite shape. All that is observable around us compels us to the conclusion that, repeatedly, over the vast expanses of time, profound and extremely sudden changes have occurred in the structure of plants and animals. Similarly, every active being, strives towards its fulfillment by turning points in its life — not by gradual evolution. These changes are of a cosmic origin and are beyond human comprehension.

Along with each new genus form is associated a definite energy by virtue of which it keeps itself pure and strong or becomes dull and evasively splits into numerous varieties. Many of these varieties fall inevitably to extinction.

What has unfolded on this blue planet is an ever-increasing richness of organic form comprising the great classes of living things which exist aboriginally and exist still — without any transition types.

The human life-form, like every other, originated in a sudden mutation of which the essential "when," "how," and "why" remains an impenetrable secret.

One thing is known, after the discovery of fire, the fate of the human animal and the entire planet was altered forever.

The origins of cooking are obscure. Primitive humans (Homo erectus, Neanderthal, and Homo sapien) may first have tasted roast meat by chance and curiosity, when the flesh of a beast killed in a forest fire was found to be more palatable and easier to chew and digest than raw meat. They probably did not deliberately cook food, though, until 500,000 years ago, after they had learned to use fire for light and warmth. Homo erectus, such as "Peking man," roasted meats, including human flesh.

The human tribes that were able to control fire eventually mastered those without that technology. Thus fire, as a technology, spread throughout the old world with fire reaching some races, such as the Africans, only 40,000 years ago.

At the same time, humans, being a curious species, experimented with cooked foods and unwittingly became addicted to them. There is a lesson to be learned here about technology's dual nature.

From cookery's beginnings some 500,000 years ago (probably in northern Europe or Asia), roasting spitted meats over fires remained virtually the sole culinary technique for several hundred thousand years. It was when human tribes became addicted to cooked animal flesh that the hunter/gatherer mode of life arose. As humans became weaker from cooked food, they became less resistant to the elemental forces of Nature and thus the need for clothing and sheltered living, such as cave dwelling, began. Present evidence suggests that the first definite cave occupations coincided with the controlled use of fire. Before fire, humans lived an advancing, frugivorous, agricultural existence in harmony with Nature's intent and design.

Cooking became more severe in the late Paleolithic Period, when tribes, such as the Aurignacian people of southern France, began to steam their food over hot embers by wrapping it in wet leaves. Aside from such crude procedures as toasting wild grains on flat rocks and using shells, skulls, or hollowed stones to heat

liquids, no further culinary advances were made until the introduction of pottery during the Neolithic Period.

The earliest compound dish was a crude paste (the prototype
of the pulmentum of the Roman legions and the polenta of later
Italians) made by mixing water with the cracked kernels of wild
grasses. This paste, toasted to crustiness when dropped on a hot
stone, made the first bread.

Technological advances notwithstanding, cookery today is
basically what it has been since Neolithic times. People still
roast, grill, and bake their foods, using dry-heat techniques
known, at least in rudimentary form, for countless millennia.
They still sauté food in small amounts of fat, fry food in deep
fat, boil food in liquids, and stew and braise food in lesser
amounts of liquid, as people have done since the development of
pottery.

Unfortunately, after the discovery of fire Homo sapiens'
natural evolution has stopped, and what is worse, it is retrogress-
ing at an incredible pace (just as it had for Homo erectus and
Neanderthal before us — both sub-species cooked their food).
Most of the Homo sub-species and races that had mastered fire
are now extinct. Cooked food has genetically damaged the still
surviving races of Homo sapien. Just imagine everyone as they
would appear nude. The vast majority of humanity is debased,
deformed, and unfit to continue the next step in evolution.

Fire-processing and other ridiculous means of food degeneration have been entirely overlooked by all anthropologists in
their study of human evolution and yet it is *by far* the most
important item to study. The whole idea that cooked food is
natural or normal is based upon a massive assumption. Cooking
is preternatural; it exists outside of Nature. It fills the body with
dead, lifeless material, stale water, flaccid cells, it allows microbes to go uncontrolled, creates disease, but worst of all,
cooked food divorces humanity from its instincts and causes
unnatural behavior in the species. All this, while raw-eating is
Nature's most patent truism, observable and demonstrable any-
where, anytime.

There are billions of species of living creatures in this vast
world. They have neither doctors, nor hospitals, nor pharmacies,

yet — with the exception of those that are under human care — they live without succumbing to illnesses and complete their proper span of life, corresponding to their environments and physical constitutions, varying from a few minutes to hundreds of years. Because of the advanced structure of the body, Homo sapiens should enjoy a longer and healthier life than most creatures on Earth.

Animals typically live six to eight times their maturation age. Carnivores fall on the shorter end and herbivores fall on the longer end of the spectrum. Horses mature in three years and often live up to 24 years. It is generally agreed that Homo sapiens mature by the age of 21 years. So humans, living naturally, should live up to an age of 120 to 170 years. There have been documented cases of people living beyond 120, even up to 150 years of age, simply by living under natural conditions away from civilization, where the extreme degeneration of foods is avoided. The very fact that most people live shortened life spans is a clear indication that something is wrong with their way of life. In the earliest periods of the world's history, the lives of the inhabitants were more youthful and perfect. These primitive humans had gigantic size, incredible strength, and a most astonishing life span. You are now living in an age where conditions are almost incompatible with longevity.

What is it that distinguishes human beings from an animal if not their habit of nourishing themselves according to the laws of "civilization" and then sitting at their desks leisurely in some artificial cave, with artificial lighting, and artificial hot or cold air circulating about the room? Picture to yourself what it would be like if one day a herd of deer decided to eat their fodder after boiling it in a cauldron and, on becoming ill, to pretend that the reasons were unknown. Would they be able to escape their predators on a diet of cooked food? Would they be able to survive the harsh, cold winters? If someone suggested that they ought to try nourishing themselves on raw grass they would become superstitious and fearful. After all, raw grass might harm them because they are now "adapted" to eating cooked food. Picture to yourselves, too, what these deer would look like today if they had consumed cooked grass for thousands of years. Yet this is precisely the position that today's narrow-minded cooked-food worshippers have placed themselves in.

Always in denial, cooked-foodists are quick to point out that "humans are carnivorous because tribes of chimpanzees hunt and eat animals." A span of six million years separates humans (Homo sapien) from chimpanzees (Pan troglodyte). Since chimpanzees are humanity's closest genetic relatives then "humans must be meat eaters too." This logic begs a closer analysis.

First, only forest-dwelling chimps engage in hunting behavior, unlike their savannah relatives. They typically hunt once a week, sometimes more, and one kill is spread throughout the adults of the tribe. So, raw meat comprises a very small percentage of their overall diet.

Secondly, massive physiological evidence exists that indicates humans and chimpanzees are frugivorous animals (see Appendix B). Chimpanzees eat leaves with bactericidal properties immediately after consuming raw flesh to aid in the unnatural digestion of flesh. Eating small animals is contrary to the frugivorous biological design of the chimpanzee. Thus they fall victim to parasitic diseases. Chimps mature in seven years and thus should live between 42 and 56 years. Meat-eating chimpanzees never make it past the age of 35.

Thirdly, chimpanzees are strong enough to hunt without any natural predation tools. Humans would not be able to catch and kill anything without tools. Do you have it in your psychological and physiological make-up to hunt down an animal, take it down in the wild, barefoot, with no clothes or technology? Yet it is without shoes, clothes, and technology that humans lived for millions of years.

In essence, chimpanzees are intelligent enough to engage in social hunting behavior they were not instinctively designed for, just like humans. Humans have taken it one step further, however, by cooking. Fortunately, chimpanzees have enough sense not to cook flesh before eating it.

Cooked food is poison.

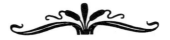

Chapter 22

The Basis For All Vices And Addictions

*"Where green life has been effectively
extinguished, in inner-city ghettos and prisons,
mental illness and violence are commonplace."*
— **Ann Wigmore**

Eating raw eradicates all other vices, such as alcoholism, all types of smoking, drug addiction, and unnatural behaviors. These vices can no more accompany raw-eating than a lion can kiss a lamb. These vices are the satellites of cooked-food addiction. *Cooked food is the first and worst addiction. It is the physio-chemical basis for all other addictions.*

Diseased bodies produce diseased minds. With improper diet the brain creates distorted representations of the world's reality.

All of humanity's ridiculous habits find their basis in cooked food. For example, the touch of skin is an indispensable part of living. To completely develop physiologically and psychologically, children need to be held and touched. Clothing must not interfere with the process. Indeed, clothing best serves to hide the abominable physical deformities in modern wo/men caused by denatured food. Rubber soled shoes electrically insulate you from the Earth, further increasing your isolation from Nature. Human beings have become cooked-carnivorous mutants. If your god had meant us to be nude, we would have been born that way!

Drug addictions are based on cooked food. The most effective means of destroying a drug habit is to eliminate cooked food from the diet, for this wipes out the basis for the addiction. What people do not realize is that a 100% raw-food diet is actually the greatest "high" in the world. Cooked-foodists resort to intoxicating substances and beverages because somewhere deep down they realize something is wrong, thus they seek to reach a natural euphoria artificially. These three authors used to drink beer and party just like most college students in America. Once we began to eat exclusively raw foods, our bodies would not allow us to even drink one beer.

Pollution begins with cooked food. When you pollute your own body by eating dead, denatured food, you will inevitably pollute the Earth. As above, so below. The human body is a self-contained world with trillions of living, breathing residents. Each resident cell deserves to live a happy, healthy life free from toxins and poisons. Just look into any garbage can or take a trip out to a landfill; at least 80% of the trash is directly attributable to the commercial distribution of cooked-food products. The percentage of refuse that is indirectly attributable to cooked-food is much higher.

Overpopulation is itself a result of cooked-food addiction because cooked food irritates the sexual organs. Cooked foods, especially dead animal products, push people through puberty early. The organism constantly wants to reproduce, because it is getting signals that it is dying by the destroyed food coming in.

People with uncontrollable, unnatural sexual desires, such as child molesters, rapists, and nymphomaniacs, are notoriously known to have the most unnatural, cooked diets. How much more obvious can it be? (And for psychiatrists and surgeon generals who may believe that masturbation is normal: There is absolutely nothing normal about male humans ejaculating for no reason.)

All of humanity's ghastly inclinations, those dark sides of animal behavior, are multiplied a thousand-fold by cooked-food addiction. Cooked food enslaves people to their most base passions.

It is cooked-food addiction that breeds all the dysgenic wars and massacres in the world. It is cooked-food addiction that brings into existence monsters like Stalin, Churchill, and Roosevelt, who, filled with the fury of greed and ambition, dare to destroy whole nations by carpet-bombing beautiful cities filled with innocent wo/men and children.

It is cooked-food addiction that gives birth to such brutal criminals as Leon Trotsky (Bronstein), whose Russian Revolution butchered some 30 million people and drove other countless millions out of their ancient homeland, where they had lived for thousands of years, robbing and pillaging their plows and their spades, their cows and their sheep, their homes and their farms, their mountains and their valleys, and then shamelessly parading before the eyes of the whole "civilized" world with complete impunity.

Should, by some impossible twist of fate, the whole world come to its senses and adopt a raw-food diet, there would be no untimely deaths during the next three or four decades, until some people reached extreme old age (barring accident, of course). As it is, the deaths caused by cooked-eating exceed, by thousands of times, all the deaths incurred in all the wars combined throughout history.

By the abolition of cooked-eating people's passions will calm down and relax, their minds will be ennobled; childbearing will be easy; life will become carefree — not some mad dash for the most material pleasures. After the victory of raw-foodism, pollution, and the dysgenic population explosion will end. Indeed all the infamous crimes against Nature will cease.

What everything boils down to is poison — sheer addiction.

Raw spelled backwards is War. If we don't get together and war on pollution, we all perish. War for life.

Cooked food is poison.

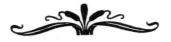

Chapter 23

Nutrition Is No Science

"Science is always simple and profound.
It is only half-truths that are dangerous."
— Bernard Shaw

In the realm of philosophy people know nothing, but in the realm of nutrition, people know less than nothing.

One hundred percent raw-eating is the only way to free humanity from dysgenesis, degeneration, and disease. Moderation has no meaning when all cooked foods are harmful. Half-measures have never and will never achieve the desired results. All the accepted calculations concerning the nutritive values of specific diets are erroneous and must be dispensed with. No matter what illness someone suffers from or what diet one practices, the only distinctions that have any meaning are raw versus cooked, Nature versus unnature. The recommendations made every day through the mass media on the use of specific vitamins, minerals, proteins, fats, and the information given on their caloric value are totally hypothetical, worthless, and dangerous — especially when they are based on the use of artificial drugs and animal products.

People must not concern themselves with the properties of individual nutritive substances, such as specific vitamins or minerals. It is the undiminished presence of all the various constituents in every bite of food that must be compulsory. None of these constituents should be absent in any of the foods people consume and this can only be assured by eating raw plant foods.

Nobody knows for certain how many different elements constitute a grape or any other fruit. Let us assume an approximate number, say: six million. By the most elementary Laws of Nature we should then have to reason that the raw materials necessary for the human organism are composed of six million different substances, and in supplying those materials it is important to take particular care that none of the constituents are absent. This is the most natural system for ensuring the normal operation of the human organism.

The dietetics of this cooked world boggle the mind. This is an age in which there are $1,000,000 prizes awarded to the baker of the finest cake, while the farmer who grows the largest or best vegetable is usually given a blue ribbon and a picture in the local newspaper. Human beings carry on the mass destruction of essential foods and nourish their bodies with only a few varieties of their debased elements.

After years of painstaking research, biologists find that there are only one thousand substances in cheese, liver, fat, or animal muscle. One would have expected them to confess that as a result of their long labor they have found that such-and-such foodstuffs consist of only a 1,000 debased, unbalanced, poison-bearing, degenerate, and dead substances and that, of the constituents forming our raw materials, 5,999,000 varieties are absent and therefore those foodstuffs are so deficient, harmful, and dangerous that their use as edibles must not be recommended by anybody to anyone.

But instead, they specify one by one the names of all the substances that they have managed to find in those dead foods. They describe in detail their functions in nutrition. After enumerating their properties, they recommend them as "beneficial" nutriments. Not once do they mention the absence of those millions of nutritive constituents, nor do they speak of their role in nutrition, or of the disastrous results that invariably follow their absence. Yet these considerations are quite essential aspects of the question.

It must be born in mind that so manifold are the functions of raw foodstuffs in the organism that even if by some miracle humans came to know them all, an entire lifetime would not suffice just to describe them. You must regard as one of the elementary laws of nutrition the fact that no nutritive constituent can serve its true purpose if it is taken in isolation, apart from the whole.

When one points out to even the most famous scientist that there is no trace of any vitamins in the bread which s/he eats, s/he retorts, without the least hesitation, that s/he also eats foods containing vitamins. With equal justification a bricklayer may lay bricks all day long and raise a wall without any mortar, and then argue that there are times when s/he uses mortar, too. Such is the blindness that is caused by cooked-food addiction.

What is bread if not starch, sugar, fats, proteins, and several types of corrosive salts - in other words, only the lifeless ashes of a few of the six million constituents forming your raw materials? What is refined sugar if not one of the above six million? What is cooked meat if not poison-containing proteins and traces of a few degenerated constituents? Yet humans fill their stomachs to the brink with these few substances and deprive their organs of millions of really essential nutriments. As to the resulting disorders that come about in their organs, one may form an idea by visiting hospitals or examining the illustrations in medical text-books. How could such terrible deformations, sores, and ulcers be caused, if not through the absence of superior nutrients?

Although scientists have so far discovered only a thousand or so types of nutritive elements, they devote large sections of medical literature to the description of the effects of those substances. These supposed effects form the basis of a great deal of other medical activities. Thus today, a vast net of commercial establishments has spread throughout the length and breadth of the world for the manufacture and distribution of those substances.

Human beings have lost sight of the integrity of the real raw materials needed for their bodies. Either people believe they are not immediately at their disposal or they find it impossible to obtain them. So they have to look into every commercial or pharmaceutical recommendation to find them — one by one — in order to satisfy their perceived needs.

Research scientists regard as scientific only those substances whose formulae are known to them and are printed in books. As they have no knowledge of the complete formulae of the constituents of a grain of wheat, they do not see anything scientific in it. It is a "common" substance that is easily obtainable, abounds everywhere, and is known to everybody. But it is quite a different matter when they succeed in discovering a new nutritive constituent and determine its formula. It then becomes scientific; its discovery is hailed as a great triumph in the field of medicine and, what is more, it introduces fresh fervor and enthusiasm into factories, pharmacies, and clinics. And this is all because humans do not wish to give up their precious bread.

Come what may, people must at last admit that the only way to get rid of diseases is first to limit strictly and then to prohibit altogether the mass destruction of raw plant foods.

To this end responsible bodies must engage in intensive media publicity campaigns and must take active measures to prevent the mass destruction of natural foods. They must recommend fruits, herbs, and new varieties of salads to the public, whose nutritional habits will then undergo a gradual change. As a result, the diseases that now afflict humanity will progressively be eliminated and an immense economy will be generated in the cost of living.

For literally centuries now, people have made nutrition their area of particular "expertise" and "knowledge." Because they have focused on only secondary problems and have not taken into consideration the preposterous nature of the kitchen fire, their research has completely failed to produce the desired results. In fact, due to their enormous contradictions, their recommendations have been a disaster.

Even vegans, who may be regarded as some of the most progressive of peoples, have not only tolerated the self-destruction inherent in the kitchen fire, but they have also put up with the use of loathsome breads and refined sugars — which are devoid of all valuable qualities. Nevertheless, it must be admitted that in the conquest of human addictions, vegans have passed several tests. Abstinence from meat and dairy products is a great step that opens the way for the conquest of breads and pastas. Vegans, and other types of vegetarians, must combine their efforts under the banner of raw-foodism in order to lay the foundation for a saner world.

Nutrition is basic and simple and does not require special "expertise" or "knowledge." Dietetics is a fraud. Only one thing is needed. The entire world must be thoroughly acquainted with the fact that eating cooked food is an addiction and that raw plant food is the only real nourishment. Humanity's present, self-immolating feeding habits are in need of a radical change. The prescription of special diets and pills must cease.

Any true scientist knows that no person who feeds exclusively on bread, rice, or cooked meat can hope to live long. But ordinary people do not realize this; some actually believe they are receiving excellent nourishment. The forces of addiction are so strong that cooked-foodists often cannot help but overdose on these abominable foods — they know no better. Even some of society's most eminent people are unable to resist the addictive urges of those vile substances and eventually fall victim to diabetes, cancers, and strokes.

It is not merely sufficient to propagate these ideas in books; it is also necessary to mobilize the proper media outlets in order to at least inform people of the facts, so that they might make an intelligent choice. Active measures must eventually be taken to eradicate the massive waste of complete plant foods and to encourage their undefiled consumption. The final objective of every kind of diet is raw-foodism. The word "(die)t" will eventually lose its meaning and be replaced simply by "natural nutrition."

Cooked food is poison.

Chapter 24

Humans Need Little Nourishment

"Death cannot feed Life."
— Jay Kordich, "The Juiceman"

The relative quantities of natural nutritive elements in whole foods vary greatly. For every milligram of one substance there may be a thousandth of a milligram of a second substance and a six millionth of a milligram of a third substance. But the substance weighing one six millionth of a milligram is just as essential for the proper functioning of the human organism as that weighing one milligram. During cooking and baking, it is precisely those substances that exist in small traces which are completely destroyed.

Many people wonder why, with such defective building materials, the human organism does not immediately stop functioning. The human body continues its operations for quite a long time, thus leading people to the erroneous conclusion that the human digestive system can adapt to anything and that it is perfectly acceptable to turn it into a toxic waste dump.

How can people live 100% cooked for months at a time and yet manage to stay alive? The answer is two-fold.

First, even the most horrible cooked-food addict takes in some raw nourishment, albeit haphazardly (e.g., iceberg lettuce on a cheeseburger). The differentiated cells may starve for weeks or months, but because fruits and vegetables are exceedingly condensed and highly-nourishing foods, a very small quantity of them keeps those cells alive. But if that starvation is exceedingly prolonged (for the cooked-foodist does not feel this hunger), various disorders such as skin sores, even scurvy, appear in the organism, not to mention the behavioral disorders that are always present among 100% cooked-food people.

Second, Nature has been very indulgent to humankind. The human organism is an incredibly flexible organic machine. It is an enormous ocean with trillions of inhabitants, innumerable enzymatic systems, various structural organizations, untold reserves, etc. Even if an individual does not receive any nutrition at all, one can survive up to 100 days and beyond by calling up stored-up nutrients and drawing in energy out of the air and rays from the sun. The raw-foodist Barbara Moore, who walked across the United States in forty-six days at the age of fifty-six, has explained that she could spend three months in the mountains of Switzerland and Italy surviving on air and snow alone. The human animal is a much different creature than most have been led to believe.

Although the human body is very flexible, it can only take so much.

What has happened is that the different human races have developed a range of tolerance to cooked foods — just like a tolerance built up against alcohol over time. This tolerance doesn't stop the damage, however, it just delays the effects. Cooked food continues to wreak both apparent and genetic havoc right into the last age of life, when the addiction consumes the whole person and entangles the true body in the firm coils of death.

In reality, cooked-foodists owe their entire existence to those few raw nutrients that they sometimes eat haphazardly. They never take into account their true importance. Because the human organism can maintain its existence on an unbelievably small quantity of nourishment, those small amounts of raw nutriments suffice to keep an individual alive for quite some time.

One must look deeper into the digestive process to see the egregious short and long-term consequences of improper feeding. After entering the digestive canal, the nutrients in food are distributed via the blood throughout the body; each cell, having an affinity for certain substances, receives its allotted share. But the specialized cells of the glands and organs take nothing from the degenerated elements present in cooked food. So those highly-developed cells must keep on waiting, in hunger and deprivation, until the organism decides to eat a berry fruit, a seeded vegetable, or a green, leafy herb.

People do not feel the starvation of normal individual cells on the conscious level, notwithstanding the extreme hunger of the differentiated cells, because their stomach is full, their addiction satisfied, their hunger abated. Their satisfaction is bolstered by the contentment felt by the growing worthless, indolent, and inactive cells, which greedily devour each "fully-balanced" meal.

Within the body, disease has mass which is often mistaken for "strength and bulk." This is why (even with 50 kilograms of surplus, useless cells) so-called "healthy, stout, and vigorous" people often lack even a few hundred grams of active, specialized cells by which their glands and organs may function properly. The ease at which their bones are broken or ligaments torn or muscles pulled is a true testament to the deficiency of living vitamins and minerals in their diet. As long as the glands and organs have not been deprived of those last remnants of active cells, people are able to drag on their existence somehow; but when those cells are at last spent, death is inevitable. *Those people truly die of starvation — cellular starvation.*

The common problem of heart starvation occurs when the heart cells lose the necessary energy and elasticity to make normal contractions. The heart then tries to save the situation by increasing the number of its cells, as a result it becomes enlarged with cells formed from cooked meat, cheese, and bread. But this is of no avail, because these cells lack the capacity to perform any essential work; it doesn't take long before the coronary artery clogs up and the heart stops beating altogether.

Cooked food is poison.

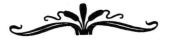

Chapter 25

The Basic Experiment

"I have steadily endeavored to keep my mind free so as to give up any hypothesis however much beloved, as soon as facts are shown to be opposed to it. Indeed, I have had no choice but to act in this manner."
— **Charles Darwin**

The principles of raw-foodism must first be adopted within the families of well-thinking people and then in the nurseries, homes for children and the elderly, prisons, and hospitals of the present age. They should then be popularized by means of a massive onslaught of media publicity. With such plain and irrefutable facts as we have presented, it is to be hoped that clear-sighted individuals will set to work at once.

The truth does not fear investigation. If people wish to have further concrete proofs, we propose the following test: Let the terminally ill in one of the world's hospitals be divided into two equal groups, one of which should be fed by current medical guidelines, the other fed by the principles of raw-foodism. Then let the health of the two groups be compared with each other over time. We have no doubt whatsoever that right from the beginning it will be clear to the whole world which of the two systems of nutrition is truly scientific and humane.

The warden of the Louisiana State Penitentiary — the largest prison in the United States — has said that prisoners age 20 percent faster because of the food they are served (high in animal fats, lifeless starches, etc.). And he says this without the slightest inkling of the raw-food/cooked-food information.

What better place to start with the cleansing activity of raw-foodism than behind the cement walls of your country's prisons? Surely upon knowing that their lives are withering away faster because of the absolute slop they are fed, even the most mentally unsound prisoners would volunteer for such an experiment. Who knows? Maybe all it takes for complete rehabilitation of a prisoner is the will to live in harmony with Nature, not against it. Rehabilitation is virtually impossible with cooked-food poisons ravaging through one's body creating violent homicidal impulses, especially in an environment of cement and iron with no trees.

In the late 1940s, in California, Jay Kordich, known to the world as "The Juiceman," conducted one such experiment on prisoners suffering from ulcers. Working with sixty-five stomach ulcer sufferers, he began treatment with cabbage juice, which is saturated with the amino acid glutamine. Within a few weeks, all but two patients were completely cured and the two laggards had only minimal symptoms. Of course, it would have taken much less time if the patients had eaten only cabbage. Who knows what else they were eating at the time of the experiment? The process of juicing raw plant food contradicts our philosophy of eating raw foods in their natural state, but extreme situations require extreme measures. Sometimes it is necessary to use every bit of technology, such as a juicer or blender, that is at your disposal.

Here is another possible experiment: Take a bum off the street and force feed her raw fruits and vegetables. Let us just see what happens.

Many ignorant people may object to the above described experiment on the ground that it is sinful or injurious to carry out such "tests." However, if such people were able to think a little deeper, they would see that it is not an experiment to safeguard life and health with the raw plant foods intended by Nature as humanity's exclusive nourishment. The real experiments are those inhumane tests that are conducted under the guise of science. The most innocent children are indiscriminately fed cooked foods and synthetic substances barely recognized in the laboratory. As a result of this, millions of children depart from life in their infancy, leaving their parents behind in bitter grief. Experiments are those operations that play with a person's health.

It is simply the unwitting ingestion of a thousand-and-one degenerated foodstuffs and poisons which creates new diseases. We have named them "the diseases of civilization," but they are really the diseases of ignorance, superstition, and unwholesome savagery.

Cooked food is poison.

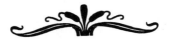

Chapter 26

Raw-Food: The Bridge To Higher Humanity

*"Watch and listen you solitaries! From the future
come winds with a stealthy flapping of wings;
and good tidings go out to delicate ears.
You solitaries of today, you who have seceded from
society, you shall one day be a people: from you, who
have chosen out yourselves, shall a chosen people spring
— and from this chosen people, the Superhuman.
Truly, the Earth shall yet become a house of healing!
And already a new odour floats about it, an odour
that brings health — and a new hope!"*
— **Friedrich Nietzsche**, *Thus Spoke Zarathustra*

We have proposed a radical and at the same time a very
simple and natural method by which humankind will be freed
from every illness. This is a very important matter to which all
scientists, doctors, intellectuals, and responsible state authorities
must give immediate attention. They must either prove publicly
that we are wrong and refute our views by fundamental experiments, or they must confirm their truth and take the necessary
steps to put them into practice. In particular, should any indifference or silence be exhibited by doctors, it may be construed
by the general public as a clear case of unwillingness on their
part to ward off diseases, in order that their sphere of activities
and cash flow may not be reduced. Doctors must give positive
proof that they have a nobler aim than the making of money, and
that their objective is, in fact, service to science and humanity.

Noble, public-spirited, and altruistic doctors reach their
aspired objective by the acceptance of raw-foodism, whereas
inhuman, selfish, and covetous doctors see in it their loss. *The
alleged difficulty of changing deep-rooted customs can only serve*

as a flimsy excuse to veil the miserly self-interests of wicked, cooked people.

Unfortunately, most doctors are really salespeople. They are merely selling people an imaginary right to escape the consequences of their actions. Doctors only know how to use technology to diagnose and prolong the miserable lives of cooked-eaters.

There is no activity of greater human value than the propagation of raw-foodism. It is necessary to awaken all humankind from its eon-old slumber, to shake it out of its lethargy, and to free it from its present nightmare. The rich must donate their money to this cause; the intellectuals their brains.

It is necessary to form societies, establish clubs, publish journals, and print books. Furthermore, it is requisite to construct spacious sanitoria with all the amenities for rest, entertainment, and sports. At these sanctuaries people can spend a few months healing, rejuvenating, and relaxing free from the destructive tendencies of society. These places will help and enlighten those people who lack the necessary information and will-power. It is much more useful and desirable to devote money and energy to this purpose than to construct churches, build synagogues, establish schools, and multiply hospitals.

Raw-foodism is the bridge which can carry humanity out of its degeneration and decay. It is an absolute prerequisite for any type of eugenics program. Raw-foodism brings forth a new kind of genius; a genius bred for self-mastery (the connection between breed and self-mastery has always been significant); a genius who has discovered how to increase the intensity of thought to the point where s/he can freely communicate with sources of knowledge not available through ordinary channels; a genius to restore this planet's vitality.

Raw-foodism is a touchstone by which we may verify which intellectual is really in possession of free and unfettered judgment, or which responsible government official or racial leader is indeed interested in the health and well-being of their people. It is in letters of platinum that time will record the names of such people.

Cooked food is poison.

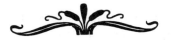

Chapter 27

We Are Not Milquetoast

*"It may be mere chance that I have never met
an honest pacifist... I have never heard of any
pacifist organization that will face facts."*
— Ezra Pound

We hold it as self-evident that a doctrine which does not attack and affect the life of the era in its inmost depths is no doctrine at all and had better not be taught.

Some people accuse us of being too extreme; too fanatical in our approach. When we call cooked-eaters murderers, filicides, and criminals, we are not making accusations; we are merely telling the truth, as bitter as that truth may be. We are militant raw-foodists. We are not here to tickle your ears with milquetoast rhetoric like some insincere politician. We are objective truth-seekers and we put forth that truth completely undiluted and pure. When a mother fills the mouth of her beloved child with hot food, she impairs the organs of her child by her own careful hands and leads it to illness and death. When a doctor prepares a diet of "nutritious" and "easily digestible" meals for small children and prescribes artificial vitamin pills at the expense of vegetables and fruits, s/he commits an even greater offense.

Every day we observe how, by a strange irony of fate, the weak and the diseased regard as curative those very substances that have been the cause of their illnesses, and devour them greedily, while on the contrary, they shun with fright the only substances (raw plant food) that can restore them to health, because they regard them as the cause of their afflictions. Millions of lives are sacrificed solely because of this fatal misconception. *The person who penetrates the full depth of the tragedy can never remain silent.*

We come across powerfully because our information needs to shock people out of their lethargic indifference. We are super-heroes and our job is to save lives. Success for us means sharing our insight and experience with others. If we help others, they will not unwittingly perpetuate cooking's self-destructive cycle.

Although any amount of raw food is better than every amount of cooked food, a 100% raw-food diet is the only normal and natural way to live. *There is one radical solution to humanity's insane war against Nature — 100% raw-eating.* The solution to the world's problems has been found. The problem is people are terrified of the answer or cannot believe its simplicity.

Henceforth, it is the foremost duty of all progressive thinkers, scientists, doctors, entrepreneurs, writers, and philanthropists to demonstrate to the general public every aspect of the enormous damage done to all life-forms by humanity's cooked-food addiction. They must exhort people to unconditionally obey the Laws of Nature.

We are not the least bit concerned with human law. Just think that, in America, it is a crime to grow marijuana — a plant; but poisoning millions of people through toxic foods is business as usual. Politics and economics are the cooked excrement of human thought. Instead of creating laws to impose false and artificial order upon humanity, laws must be based on the order of life. Natural laws require little explanation; their meaning is irrevocable in its simplicity and specificity.

Only those who have completely surpassed their desire for cooked food can experience the highest forms of life, not the mundane life of the mortal, but the divine life of the resurrected.

Those who are afraid to look at the philosophy of Raw-foodism are revealing how cowardly and bourgeois they really are.

We give a clear signal to our enemies that we intend to be hostile. We give no quarter and show no mercy.

Cooked food is poison.

Chapter 28

Take Action

"Nature is no sentimentalist, it does not cosset or pamper us. We must see that the world is rough and surly, and will not mind drowning a man or a woman, but swallows your ship like a grain of dust."
— **Ralph Waldo Emerson**

"Procrastination, or the inability to take action, is the number one reason for failure."
— **Napoleon Hill**

When a slight defect comes to light in the proper balance of the raw materials supplied to the industry of a country, the individuals responsible are accused of negligence and reprimanded, whereas those who commit the most hideous adulteration in the raw materials necessary for the proper workings of the human organism, often go unnoticed. In the present age of scientific advance the most ignorant and stupid person has the absolute right to look for new methods of degenerating natural foodstuffs, and to concoct and offer for sale the most ridiculous eatables.

What is particularly strange is the fact that the great scientists, the great cytologists, who have devoted their lives to the study of the biological functions of the living cells, or the dietitians, whose primary aim in life is the working out of the ideal diet for human beings, purchase, en masse, such degenerated substances. They offer them to their own cells, with the utmost indifference and carelessness, guided by the dictation of their palates alone.

Provided that the cells of a gland or organ are not wholly spent, natural nutrition enables them to restore their essential

complement of cells by giving birth to new cells and by eliminating diseased and useless cells. There is no means at all of
returning an ashen organ, such as a decayed tooth, to its former
state. That is why, in matters of health, procrastination is
dangerous.

The philosophy of natural nutrition is so sensible, that to
many people it is totally incomprehensible. At first sight it may
seem unbelievable that you could free yourself of a disease or
illness by means of raw-foodism. But the greatness of the
proposition lies in the very fact that the "unbelievable" easily
becomes an accomplished reality. Because abandoning cooked
food is instinctive and natural, it is not as difficult to do as one
might imagine — although it may take time to wean oneself from
cooked food. Once an individual reaches a certain point of
dietary advance, the body's biochemistry improves drastically
and will not allow that individual to return to decadent foods.

The supposed difficulty of relinquishing cooked-food addiction must not be regarded as an obstacle. On the contrary, it
must serve as a measure to gauge the strength of the enemy. It
must spur people on to make every effort to prevent the entry of
such an appalling monstrosity into the mouth of a newborn child.
Even those people who find it difficult to forsake cooked meals
themselves, and still persist in their harmful habits, must affirm
the truth, and for the sake of the rising generation and the future
of humankind they must fight for the victory of that truth by
teaching and expounding the principles of raw-foodism by all
other means available.

We have found that people have various desires which
motivate them.

Some are motivated by the desire to please the opposite sex.
A raw-food diet is the way to bring out your natural inner beauty
and sexual charm. It cultivates a special charisma and positive
attitude which magnetically attracts beauty into your life.

Others are motivated by their desire for revenge. Raw-
foodism is the ultimate revenge. By your enhanced attitude,
energy, and life span there is no way for others to compete with
you in the long-term. In your enemy's eyes, your grander goals,

desires, and achievements means their total failure. *Revenge is a dish best served raw.*

For some, it takes a brush with death, a tremendous fear, before they alter their habits. Fear is the mind-killer, but it is also the key to enlightenment. Often, out of desperation comes inspiration.

No matter what your age, it is not too late. You can be rejuvenated. When we see an apple entering the mouth of a child, we know that it is *never* too late — for the individual or the human species.

In the present age people want fast food to keep apace with their "busy" lives. The fastest food is a piece of fruit. What could be faster than an apple or a pear? Cooked-foodists come up with any excuse why they cannot alter their diet. Why don't they come up with excuses on why they can do it? Is it that the truth is hard to swallow? It shouldn't be, just take a handful of watermelon and shove it in your mouth.

Don't fool yourself. A smart individual is one who is honest with her/himself. Choose success instead of failure. A slight edge means everything. This is a systemless system of success — all you have to do is control what you put in your mouth. Give your body the very best, so that it can give you the very best. You can take immediate control of your mental, emotional, and physical destiny.

Of course, when a lie has gone too far, when it has surreptitiously corrupted the very brain tissue and marrow of the organism, then all remedies are useless. For those moderate and "cultured" people who are irrevocably biased in favor of cooked foods and drugs, the principles of raw-foodism are far too obvious. They always suffer an ignoble end. Nature never grants a false judgment.

Those people who are not animated by strong passions and desires are merely mediocre beings and do not deserve the splendor life has to offer. The "average person" is just that... average. Moderation is the mating call of the herd animal.

However you let this information affect you, these are self-evident truths. You will never encounter anything that matches the power of raw-foodism. Those who disagree amaze us. Everything is so logical. Everything is so natural. Any other attitude is just denial. Humanity is exhausting itself trying to fight the Laws of Nature.

People like to believe that they live in some enlightened age, but it looks to us as if they are truly in the Dark Ages, where every progressive idea or great invention is for years persecuted by the corrupt few and the ignorant masses. Today it is the question of the survival or the annihilation of the human race that is placed before humanity. Hesitation is weakness. Rise up and take action.

Cooked food is poison.

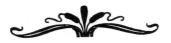

Chapter 29

Cooking: The Greatest Waste Of Resources

"Who has made the decision that sets in motion these chains of poisonings, this ever-widening wave of death that spreads out, like ripples when a pebble is dropped into a still pond?"
— **Rachel Carson**

An unbelievable quantity of nutrients is destroyed by the numerous forms of refining and processing. As an example, it may be said that one cob of raw corn has a greater nutritive value than ten bags of corn chips. The same ratio holds true when we compare all varieties of fruits and vegetables with their unnatural, cooked derivatives. If civilization dispensed with all animal foodstuffs today, the plant foods produced in the world would be able to feed, by themselves, fifty times the present population of the world, provided that they were eaten in their raw state.

The real meaning of raw-foodism will become all the more understandable, when you think of the labor, the time, and the money that people waste growing foods and then subsequently destroying them. Consider all the medical expenses incurred both by the various health institutions and by the general public in the hope of eliminating the ravages brought about in the internal organs by the destruction of those raw foods. Raw-foodism benefits the economy and raises the standard of living exponentially.

Ninety percent of the labor that it takes to plant and harvest grains, vegetables, and fruits is evaporated under the kitchen fire. Nowhere can there be found such a waste of resources — and it is all due to cooked-food addiction.

In spite of the continuous increase in the agricultural production of cereal grasses, vegetables, and fruits, there is still a great shortage of foods all over the world. There are three reasons for this strange paradox. First of all, by the process of cooking, food is deprived of all nutritional value. Then, by the help of artificial fertilization, ignorant farmers raise the quantity of the produce at the expense of its quality so they can increase their profit of produce sales to livestock raisers. Finally, the false human has been growing so rapidly that the increase in food production, so long as it has been cooked, has been quite unable to keep pace with the demand — mostly due to humanity's cooked-meat addiction.

What would it be like if the entire globe suddenly returned to a natural method of feeding? Even if agricultural production remained at its present level, every single person on the planet could have at least 10 raw fruits and vegetables a day. Most of humanity's agricultural activity goes towards feeding livestock for senseless slaughter. The amount of waste and destruction that would end instantly just by stopping the intake of animal products is beyond human comprehension — not to even mention what would happen if the kitchen fire was extinguished forever. All the labors and expenses put into the preparation of cooked food are nothing but utter waste.

All the destroyed, degenerated, and debased foods consumed by people in the world today are disposed of in three ways:

1. Due to a deficiency in the complement of specialized cells, the true body is obliged to tolerate the presence of a certain number of malformed and parasitic cells formed from dead food. An enormous quantity of cooked food is consumed by the false body.

2. The extracts are retained within the organism's intercellular fluids and cavities.

3. The redundant portion of the food which is beyond the assimilative powers of the cells is simply purged out of the system as total waste — provided, of course, that the body still has enough eliminative internal energy.

One of the most deplorable aspects of the situation is the fact that the specialized cells spend a great deal of energy they acquire from natural nutrients to break down the foods devoured by the false body. Once accumulated, those dead nutrients must be continuously pushed into the blood to be filtered and excreted.

The active cells are entitled to some rest, but cooked-foodists burden them by forcing them to work all day and night to eliminate the poisons introduced into the greedy mouth of the false body.

We are ready to demonstrate the truth of our statements by concrete proofs to anyone who may wish to have further particulars on the subject. History will never pardon those responsible people in authority who show indifference in this matter and shut their eyes and ears to these absolute truths in order to justify their personal addictions.

There can be only two reasons why authoritative people refuse to accept the principles of raw-foodism. Either they must declare that they prefer to tolerate the existence of diseases rather than to "deprive" humankind of the pleasures of cooked meals and that they prefer to maintain the "scientific achievements" attained as a result of much useless research. Or, by the performance of the basic tests proposed by us, they must prove that, far from freeing people from diseases, raw-foodism actually harms people. They will find this impossible to do. It follows that they have no alternative but to rely on their first reasoning, the extreme inhumanity which is evident to all.

Therefore, on behalf of all innocent children and animals, we demand that the opponents of raw-foodism submit their objections to the mass media, so that they may obtain a proper reply. Scientific fact-finding must have the opportunity to draw the necessary conclusions and to pronounce its final and just verdict.

Cooked food is poison.

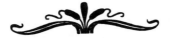

Chapter 30

Raw Materials

"Until humanity can duplicate a blade of grass,
Nature laughs at its so-called scientific knowledge."
—**Thomas Alva Edison**

Every individual is the proud possessor of the most complicated machine in the world and it is that person alone who is solely responsible for the smooth operation of that machine. It is necessary, therefore, that s/he should be thoroughly acquainted with the real, faultless, and integral raw materials that wonderful entity requires.

The integrity of raw-food materials is not determined by the quantities of proteins, fats, carbohydrates, vitamins, minerals, and calories that are specified by present-day biologists in their text-books on nutrition. Nor is it possible to determine the ideal diet by creating long lists of cooked-food recipes.

Through millions and millions of years and by the most precise calculations Nature has brought together the integral raw materials necessary for the human organism. Nature has combined them in perfect harmony and in the requisite quantities, has given them life, and has concentrated them in plant bodies in the form of living cells. The whole secret of nutrition lies in those cells being alive, not dead and dehydrated. Under no circumstances can substances consisting of dead cells serve as raw materials for the human organism.

Humanity should not lose its sense of proportion and gloat over its inventions beyond the bounds of reason. It is true that in the study of individual nutritional elements biologists have taken an immense amount of trouble and have made a great many important discoveries, which deserve some appreciation. All those achievements, however, may be regarded as great only in relation to the present technical and mental development of humanity. Against the supreme wisdom of Nature even the most eminent scientists, with all their learning and their countless discoveries, have no greater insight than a child of three. They have no right, therefore, to upset the harmony and integrity of the raw materials constructed by Nature and to impose upon the public their minuscule smattering of knowledge as perfect science.

Undoubtedly, in trying to penetrate into the secrets of food, the ultimate objective of scientists is to recognize all those nutritive elements that are essential to the human organism, to determine their relative quantities, and to integrate them together. In other words, they wish to artificially prepare a habañero pepper or a cantaloupe and give life to it. But what humanity has been unable to obtain after thousands of years of incessant labor, Nature presents to us gratuitously every day. What more do you want? Do human beings entertain any doubts concerning the wisdom of Nature or does addiction to cooked food incite them to commit the most unbelievable mistakes and blunders?

It is most senseless and dangerous to suppose that we need more proteins or other nutritional constituents than there are in plant bodies. If the latter contain only small quantities of proteins, it follows that the human organism does not need more, for it is precisely with those quantities that human organisms have been constructed and developed over a period spanning millions of years.

Some people are very fond of talking continually about body-building materials. If "fully-balanced" animal proteins and "nutritious meals" could increase the height of every generation by as little as one millimeter, today the height of humans would have increased by several meters already.

Mass-produced artificial vitamins can never serve as nutritional constituents for the very obvious reason that, quite often, within five minutes after their entry into the human body, they stop the functions of the organism altogether. In fact, they drive the human organism to death.

It is deplorable short-sightedness to regard any particular foodstuff as a source of a specific vitamin or of any other nutritive constituent. All organic compounds are formed of almost the same constituents, but they differ in their physical and chemical properties because of differences in their composition and molecular structure. Thus, everybody knows that alcohols and sugars are composed of the same chemical elements (carbon, hydrogen, and oxygen), but they differ greatly in color, taste, and appearance. Birds are imprisoned in cages with one kind of seed or grain and domestic animals are often fed on one kind of grass only. Yet these creatures obtain their full supply of proteins, fats, vitamins, and minerals from the limited foodstuffs given to them.

The treatments of disease by means of false vitamins, destructive antibiotics, and various poisons are hopeless experiments that are based not on etiological and basic reasoning, but on symptomatic, apparent, and contradictory data.

No artificial vitamin can restore the wonderful balance of those natural vitamins burned on the fire; no poison can regulate the normal biological functions of degenerated organs and glands; no antibiotic can replace the natural antibiotics destroyed in the kitchen.

Animals heal their sores by licking them. Their secretions and saliva are endowed with bactericidal and regenerative properties. The secretions of cooked-eating humans, however, are devoid of such properties. The raw-foodist wards off the danger of a serious cold through the agency of secretions released by the tissues of the respiratory tract, whereas a cooked-foodist produces streams of mucus and saliva, but is still not able to resist that very same danger.

Cooked food is poison.

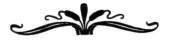

Chapter 31

Superstition And Ignorance

"Superstition? Crush the infamous thing!"
— **Voltaire**

Modern medicine is surrounded by a tangled web of vain superstitions. All medical activity is based on symptomatic, apparent, deceptive, and contradictory data, while the most essential and fundamental principle has been buried in oblivion. This principle is that the efficient operation of every machine is subject to the uniform supply of the integral raw materials specified by the engineer. In this case, the integral raw materials designed for the human machine are living plant cells and nothing else.

Intoxicated by a few technical successes, humanity today imagines itself at the zenith of civilization, while in reality, it is in a most primitive, unnatural, and gruesome state. Generally speaking, in the fields of politics, economics, morality, and health the minds and feelings of humans are ruled, and their actions directed, by loathsome addictions and vain superstitions. Forgetting the most essential and basic problems of life, humans exaggerate quite trivial matters of secondary importance and turn them into vital questions. People then waste an incredible amount of time and resources, create enmities, shed oceans of blood, pollute, and spread universal ruin for nothing more than their own pointless self-destruction.

Historians of the past have painted in the most abhorrent colors the taxes, imposts, and tributes levied by kings and foreign conquerors. Whereas today, the moment they take the helm of the state, individuals who are regarded as civilized and enlightened use various legalized pretexts to confiscate large percentages of their own peoples' earnings in order to satisfy their own short-sighted addictions and ambitions. They encourage the production of tobacco, alcoholic and non-alcoholic beverages, meat and dairy products, as well as thousands of other wares which undermine the health of the people, and then pride themselves on the increase in government income obtained from those sources.

The fact that the haphazard suggestions and recommendations found in diet books to eat more raw fruits, vegetables, and herbs do not achieve any useful results is readily apparent. Spurred on by the urge of all-powerful addictions, the nutritional habits of humankind have gradually developed a more and more frightful pattern that encourages the destruction of beautiful animals and the production of dangerous foodstuffs lacking in vitamins and minerals. Without the least rest or respite there continually arise factories for the production of smokables, alcoholic beverages, diet sodas, chips, cookies, ice cream, yogurt, canned-food, bread, butter, candy, meat, and various other dangerous substances.

The degree of human ignorance is so massive, it defies description. Obviously, citrus fruits are vital sources of living vitamins and organic minerals. In the 1750s, James Lind, a British physician, conducted one of the first reported controlled experiments in medicine. He found that sailors on long voyages without rations containing citrus fruits developed bleeding gums, rough skin, poor muscle tension, and slow-healing wounds, symptoms characteristic of the vitamin C deficiency disease called scurvy. This experiment marked the earliest proven link between a single nutrient and disease. Though Lind cured scurvy, his discovery, like most innovative ideas, went unheeded. One-hundred years later, during America's civil war, more people died of scurvy and other forms of malnutrition than of bullet wounds.

Today, things are not much different in America. The "great steak religion" has taken complete control. Each weekend a new tribute is demanded. Indeed, the chef is the religious leader of the cooked-food addict.

What kind of ignorance leads one to put a dead piece of animal muscle (steak) on a black eye?

What kind of ignorance leads one to believe that feeding their pets grapes, cantaloupe, or avocados will harm them; while feeding them factory-canned cooked meat will strengthen them?

Amongst the tangled web of humanity's fanatical presuppositions have arisen a myriad of medical misconceptions: the vitamin B-12 myth, anemia syndrome, and the protein deficiency concept are three startling examples. A vitamin B-12 deficiency arises when there is a complete disruption in the human body's intestinal flora. In a normal situation, vitamin B-12 is absorbed from bacteria in the intestinal tract. Cooked-meat eaters are not afflicted by this deficiency because, animal flesh (including insect tissue) contains a plethora of B-12. Only cooked-food vegetarians who eat extremely degenerated beverages and foods (especially carbonated soft drinks) are afflicted by a B-12 deficiency which "miraculously" disappears on a raw-food diet. If you are so worried about a B-12 deficiency, eat an insect as other primates do. Anemia is an iron deficiency which afflicts cooked-vegetarians who destroy the vitamins and minerals in their food — again this problem is easily remedied on raw food. What has been labeled a "protein deficiency" is really a set of withdrawal symptoms from cooked-meat deprivation.

All these come to prove that in the conduct of their daily life people are guided not by common sense, but by the destructive addictions and vain superstitions particular to cooked-eating humankind. There exist in this world countless political parties, religious sects, and other groups that concern themselves with trivial and secondary questions of strictly limited interest. Henceforth, the primary duty of true humanity should be to wage an urgent and decisive campaign against addictions and superstitions of every description. This is the only basic means by which humanity will succeed in attaining that plentiful, comfortable, healthy, long, and happy life which it has always desired.

Cooking stands in opposition to all intellectual well-being. It takes the side of everything idiotic. It proclaims a curse against the spirit — against the freedom of a healthy spirit. Because sickness belongs to the essence of cooking, the typical cooked-foodist mindset, filled with superstitions, has to be a form of sickness as well. *Superstition means not wanting to know what is true.*

The concrete proof is before our eyes. By means of raw-foodism not only have these three authors saved our own lives, but we have also freed ourselves from all those illnesses and unnatural behaviors that used to torment us every so often. We have completely driven away the haunting spectre of early death. The three of us, in our late twenties, have regained the health, strength, vigor, and energy of young children. For months now our days are busy and exhilarating, twenty-hours awake, working and playing, without experiencing the least feeling of weariness. We are quite sure that we shall live for one or two more full spans of a cooked-eater's life.

It seems that on some subconscious level humans realize what is going on. That is why images of "evil" are associated with fire, while images of "good" are associated with trees and sky.

In Greek mythology the titan Prometheus met his downfall when he stole fire from Olympus and shared the "gift" of fire with humanity. Appropriately, Prometheus literally means "before thinking" because he did not think before he acted. His brother, Epimetheus, literally translates into "after thinking" because he would act only after thinking of the consequences, and this is precisely what should be done every time humans employ the technology of fire.

Socrates said that human beings should eat to live and not live to eat. Now the time has come to prove who are those that regard eating as a means to an end and not an end in itself. Let such people follow our example, step into the arena, join together in a common cause, fight against every human addiction, and open up the road to a new and happy life for all humankind.

The subjects discussed in this book are not specialized questions that ought to be discussed behind closed doors. They are matters that concern humanity as a whole and must be considered publicly so that everybody may be able to recognize the real raw materials designed for the human organism.

It is the duty of all those people who are interested in the health of themselves and their children to raise their voice and demand that those who oppose the principles of raw-foodism should submit their criticisms to the mass media and prominent scientists, in order that we may have the opportunity to give them appropriate replies and thus to dispel the skepticism of the general public towards the doctrine of raw-foodism.

Cooked food is poison.

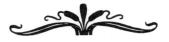

Chapter 32

We Appeal To Humanity As A Whole

"If we don't stand together, we stand to lose the future."
— Geoff Tate

The subjects that we discuss in this book are not specialized problems. They are questions which touch humanity as a whole. They affect all those who live, eat, and breathe. That is why we always try our best to write in as simple a language as possible, basing our conclusions upon general data and arguments, without clogging our writing with such scientific details and indigestible terminology as are beyond the comprehension of the majority of people. In our arguments we do not rely upon the multitude of apparent and contradictory data obtained by imperfect laboratory tests or upon any erroneous assumptions underlying such data. The proofs that we present are the irrefutable Laws of Nature. We forward such general conclusions as are obtained by basic experience, and which every individual in every corner of the globe can readily test and verify for themselves.

In reality, the concept of raw-foodism is so basic that it can be summed up in two sentences: Nature has created all foods the human organism requires — these are living fruits, vegetables, and herbs. Provided that those raw materials are ingested wholly intact, the human organism will complete its natural life span without succumbing to any illnesses.

Anybody who has a strong enough character to understand these two sentences can easily discern the deplorable state of humanity's feeding habits. It is plain to see that combatting disease with cooked foods and medicines is both erroneous and dangerous. All those methods developed by doctors have very little to do with the fundamental cause of diseases.

After years of in-depth study and intuitive personal experience, we have no doubt whatsoever that the natural system of nutrition frees humanity from all kinds of diseases. Natural nutrition guarantees for every human being a wonderfully long life filled with laughter, contentment, and comfort.

The present age of "civilization" and "progress" is a terrible nightmare, filled with pollution, addiction, and vices. Indeed, it would take six million books to fully describe all of humanity's disgusting feeding patterns and behaviors. The primary item on our agenda is for everyone to clearly understand why diseases exist and how they can be eradicated once and for all. To do this it is essential that we describe how the human organism is constructed and naturally fed.

It seems certain that life made its first appearance on the planet in the form of organelles and then later, single-celled organisms. One may picture an ameoba, which is one of the most primitive unicellular organisms on the planet. Amoebas operate independently by looking for food particles, ingesting and digesting them, excreting waste, and reproducing by mitosis.

As time passed, some of these single-celled organisms began to cooperate to form multi-cellular organisms. These complex cells abandoned the aimless life of detached amoebic individualism and grouped themselves together in more efficient communal systems where each cell adopted a particular function to perform in the creature's aggregate life. This initial cooperation of a few cells eventually developed into more and more complex arrangements. Ultimately living creatures arose which consisted of billions, even trillions, of cells. Homo sapien is one of these creatures.

One may compare human life within any of the vast political structures of the present day with cellular life inside a multi-cellular organism. Collective organizations are so much more efficient at survival that the whole mass can be maintained, even multiply, while useless, parasitic, and degenerated individuals or cells grow uncontrolled. In any society today, one may find festering bums living amongst people of extraordinary talent and genius.

This analogy also holds true within the human body. Worthless, freeloading, weak cells carry on their sluggish existence alongside extremely useful, advanced, differentiated cells. The human body, like an enormous political state, has its various organizations which are the glands, organs, tissues, etc. Every system has its particular function from the tissues of the skin, muscle, and bones, to the tissues of the brain. Those systems carry out their functions by the simultaneous efforts of particular groups of specialized cells which direct the "worker" cells and various microbes.

Thus the body functions: the nerve cells are electrically unified by fibrous tissues so that brain commands may be communicated throughout the entire body; the muscle cells possess a contractile power that enables them to perform bodily movements and engage in heavy mechanical work; the kidney cells form a system endowed with special filters which purify the blood and drain waste urine; and the cells of the glands take the necessary raw materials from the inter-cellular fluid and convert them into hormones.

Just like successful human beings, who continually thirst for the best knowledge and then convert it into action, specialized cells go straight for the best nutrients and then convert them into useful energies for the organism. Both can survive and support the edifice for quite a long time even though things have begun to crumble beneath them. Inevitably, however, disintegration reaches the point of no return. With improper nutrients, inefficiencies, malfunctions, and deaths occur.

Certainly it would be of great interest to have complete knowledge of the cellular structure and a comprehensive understanding of all the enzymatic activities and organelle processes that go on within them. But even if by some miracle humans could penetrate into all the clandestine secrets of the cells, the information would fill not merely thousands, but at least six million volumes. Not even a raw-foodist could grasp all that material in a lifetime.

Contrary to the arrogant claims of some boastful scientists, human beings have only pierced the surface of cellular complexity. With every advance in research it has become more and more clear that even the most educated biologists understand only an infinitesimal part of the whole that still remains hidden.

Yet, deceived by a few technical successes, people imagine themselves atop a peak of scientific perfection. In reality, science has done nothing more than exploit a few natural relations. In the name of progress, human beings have extensively tampered with their own bodies. People are so gravely presumptuous that, by means of the most terrible schemes, scientists have undertaken desperately insane experiments in order to remedy the multiplicity of disorders appearing in the organism. Medical science has done nothing but experiments, and all of them have involved a massive falsification of results. If people wish to destroy themselves with medicines and medical exaggerations then so be it. But anybody who performs even one more experiment on enslaved, innocent animals has no right to life.

Scholars must descend from their ivory towers and adopt a realistic view of the world. An infinitesimally small cell, by itself, has a more complex structure than all this planet's human-made machines combined. And yet, every organ is composed of billions of such cells. Nevertheless, ordinary physicians, in their crass arrogance, imagine themselves to be specialists on those extensive systems. When physicians scribble the name of some medicine on a piece of bleached paper, they naively suppose that they can restore the disorganized functions of billions of organic systems by the prescription of a single poison.

The healer of any illness is always Nature. Only the body can heal itself — the process is automatic. But doctors are quick to ascribe any recovery to medicines unless the patient's condition worsens. In that case, doctors claim that the "illness has run its natural course and there is nothing more that could have been done." How cooked is that?

What would modern medicine have a person do when their organs begin to function irregularly? Do people actually believe that some doctor or surgeon is acquainted with all the details of the human organs in the same way that a simple inventor is familiar with all the details of their simple invention? Medical science has convinced the masses that they must resign themselves to the fickle caprices of fate or submit to crazy experiments.

Fortunately, an immediate and extremely easy method exists for every human race to rid itself of all debilitations and diseases. When an engineer designs a machine, s/he determines with minute calculation the raw materials necessary for its precise operation. As long as the design engineer's plans are followed with diligence and care, the machine operates perfectly for its allotted life span.

Just as every machine has had its design engineer, so too has every organism. Each creature has been perfectly fashioned even down to the most minute calculation and detail. Because the human body is an extremely complicated organism — an amazing ocean containing trillions of cells — its design engineer must be a wonderful entity of extraordinary talent and eternal wisdom.

Therefore, if any human being could find that engineer or, at least, obtain the instruction book for the human organism, they could undoubtedly be able to complete the normal span of life without ill health and unnatural behaviors. Moreover, those people would no longer be obliged to continue those senseless poisoning experiments which have thus far produced such "magical" results.

We submit to you that the instruction book for human health is in your hands. And the design engineer of the human body is that ingenious, immense, and ineffable life-force that surrounds every living thing. It does not have to be found, for it is everywhere and universally observable.

Cooked food is poison.

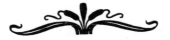

Chapter 33

Humans Are Engineered Raw

"To live simply and naturally is the highest and final goal."
— **Friedrich Nietzsche**

There can be only three reasons why a machine would break down: incidental wear and tear coming in from the outside, a flaw exists in its design, and/or a deficiency exists in the raw materials required to run the machine.

Incidental damage sustained by the human organism from external sources (burns, injuries, poisoning, etc.) are easily understood and there is no disagreement on the holistic methods to be employed in their treatments. These external damages may include all needle-administered drugs, vitamin pills, mineral supplements, alcohol, THC, tainted water, as well as those innumerable poisons introduced into the body by eating or breathing in cooked, dead, and denatured substances.

Every organism's design pattern is found in its DNA code. The genetic blueprint for the human organism has been damaged by countless millennia of unnatural feeding. The DNA code continues to be assaulted at an ever increasing pace. DNA damage is passed down from generation to generation and the flaws accumulate. With bad breeding they make their outward appearance. Genetic damage is a one-way path into an abyss from which there is no return.

The most harmonious raw materials for the human organism are the raw plant foods created by Nature. Even the slightest alteration in the type of food designed for the organism means dislocating the proper operations of the human machine — it means disease. This is an unerring axiom of Nature.

Living forces have constructed the raw materials intended for the human machine with such precise calculations that when a raspberry is placed in the mouth, it breaks up and spreads throughout the organism, fulfilling all its needs. That berry first builds the rudimentary structures of the simple cells. It then constructs all the internal machinery and mechanisms of the differentiated cells. That raspberry provides the materials necessary for cleaning and lubricating all the component parts of the organism. It renews damaged cells, replaces old and tired cells with youthful organelles. It warms the body, supplies fuel for the organism, and any other task demanded of it. Just as every design engineer specifies, through detailed calculations, the raw materials necessary for a machine, so to has Nature specified the requisite raw materials essential for humans and all other living creatures.

Nature has expended an incredible amount of energy in developing living foods for living animal organs. For simple cells, it has prepared simple building materials, which vary according to the functions of those cells. The same holds true for complex cells. Thus, the cells of the skin demand a certain type of building material, and those of the muscles require another kind. The same is true of the glands, nerves, dendritic fibers, marrow, etc. With just a touch of living energy (diatomic oxygen) the cells engage in their productive operations.

Because the human organism has an extremely intricate construction, its raw materials are of a correspondingly complex design, consisting of a myriad of organic molecules.

By its unfailing wisdom Nature has combined within the structures of living fruits, vegetables, and herbs all those raw materials required by the human organism. Each of those materials has its precise quantity. Thus, of one kind of substance, we may need a gram, of another, a thousandth of a gram. This is the operative rule for all organisms. It is essential that those materials should always be at the disposal of the cells in their predetermined ratios and quantities. Special care must be taken to insure that none of them is absent from the aggregate whole.

It is interesting to note that all living creatures, from a termite to a shark, from a mountain lion to a giraffe, recognize their natural foods and make full use of them to satisfy their nutritional needs. Paradoxically enough, humans are the only creatures to abandon their instincts and completely lose sight of those indispensable foods which are essential for their well-being. Cooked food has completely divorced humanity from its instincts.

People labor day and night in laboratories and research institutes. They conduct all kinds of useless tests and experiments to discover "natural" materials. They then manufacture them by processing raw plant foods, dead animals, or by synthesizing them artificially. Strange names are concocted for these substances. Huge multi-level marketing companies are then formed to distribute these products all over the world, so that people may be "nourished." And this is called "all-natural."

A breakfast cereal company that labels a product "100% Natural" is lying through its cooked teeth. What is natural about cooked grain? How about "0% Natural"?

Without realizing what they are doing, scientists have come into direct conflict with Nature. Blinded by addictions, these researchers are unable to see that Nature has compiled the highest forms of nutrients within countless types of fruits and vegetables. Nature has spread these all over the world, especially in the tropical zones where Homo sapien originated.

Cooked food is poison.

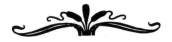

Chapter 34

All Raw Plants Are Complete Foods

"The whole is more than the sum of its parts."
— Goethe

Every mammal must eat raw plant food. All mammalian carnivores are really omnivores. Dogs must eat grass, and not just when they are ill, as popular myth dictates. Cats dig up and chew on plant roots. Brown bears typically eat 95% plant food. The reason for this is that all raw plant foods are whole. They completely nourish the body. All food chains begin with plant forms. It makes no difference what raw plant foods a species has an affinity for. What is important is that the food consumed is living, natural, and intact.

When a thoroughbred feeds on grass, nobody ever worries that the animal may suffer from an insufficiency of proteins or minerals. Animals too, like humans, need every kind of vitamin, mineral, enzyme, etc. which arise from the life-giving soil. How is it that a moose can grow into a fantastic creature on simple grass, and that a human cannot do the same on raw fruits and vegetables?

Everybody can clearly see that the food choices made by the myriad of animals that populate the Earth, consist of a limited variation. They are designed to get the foods they enjoy most and that are in their immediate vicinity. Nevertheless, we are not able to find even a single case of avitaminosis or any other nutritional deficiency among them.

If you take the foodstuffs consumed by those animals into the laboratories of biologists, in each of them they will find several substances of varying qualities and quantities. They will then tell you that in a particular plant there is so much protein, so much fat, and so much of one vitamin or another. Thus in

each plant they will enumerate some arbitrary number of constituents that they have managed to find and will carefully
determine their quantities one by one. Even in the richest fruits
the number of constituents that they have succeeded in discovering has been strictly limited. In reality, this does not prove that
each of those foodstuffs consists of only the dozen or so
constituents they have found; rather, it is an indication that their
technical skills and resources are quite inadequate to fully
analyze and to determine qualitatively and quantitatively all those
constituents that have come together in Nature's laboratory. It
means that in a particular food they have been able to discover
only those few kinds of constituents; the rest have remained
hidden from them.

The main reason for this is the fact that the substances
discovered by biologists are not the primary constituents of those
plant bodies, but they are compounds that appear in different
forms in different plant bodies. Upon entering the animal body,
those compounds are broken down to the molecular level and
synthesized again. Thus new compounds are formed corresponding to the needs of the organism.

All plant forms consumed by animals consist of the same
basic constituents. Fundamentally, all plants consist of three
main classes of substances.

The first of them is living water, which is familiar to us all.
One cannot live without water. We may well remember that the
purest and safest source of water is that found in plant bodies —
especially fruit. Plant water has been vivified and electrified by
sunlight. Humans, like all the other primates, need very little
water because their food has such a high-water content. In
Nature, we see mountain gorillas drinking by dipping a hand into
a running stream and sucking the water off the hairs on the back
of their hand. Due to the massive pollution of nearly all water
sources on the planet, one should only drink collected rain water,
eat snow, or distilled water (an unnatural creation, but useful in
extreme circumstances) if fruit or plant juice is not obtainable.
Never drink bottled spring waters in the United States because,
by law, they need only be 50% spring water, the rest can be
ordinary tap water. People drink exorbitant amounts of water to

dilute the dehydrated, cooked-food extracts which fill their bodies. Nature's reaction to internal pollution is to dilute toxic materials with water. From this logic we may conclude that Nature's reaction to external pollution is to dilute the polluted atmosphere with precipitation.

The second class consists of fiber, or roughage. This substance, cellulose, constitutes the framework of plants, giving them form and firmness. Fiber is not completely broken down and assimilated in the animal organism; it is typically expelled from the body in the form of feces. It is, however, an essential part of the animal diet. If there were no roughage in the food consumed by animals, their intestines would have nothing to expel, and in the course of time they would shrivel and dry up. Yet, many people are so short-sighted that, regarding fiber as "indigestible," they deliberately remove it from their foodstuffs, as a result of which nearly all humankind suffers from constipation. The causes of constipation are the absence of roughage in the diet and cooked-food clogging.

The last of the three classes of plant substances is the nutrient itself — the juice — which is fully digestible and can be completely assimilated by the animal organism.

The essential differences between diverse plant bodies arise from variations in the relative quantities of those three classes of substances. Thus, the main difference between the common grass and fruit is that in grass, fiber and chlorophyll predominate, whereas fruit consists of only a moderate amount of roughage, with plenty of concentrated nutriments and an adequate supply of living water. Because of the special structure of their digestive organs and their faculty of rumination, grazing herbivores are able to crush and grind the grass, to extract the nutrients dispersed in it and to expel the rest from their bodies. This is how certain animals manage to obtain nourishment from dry hay or straw; the camel is able to sustain life on desert thistles and the donkey on the roughest of grasses.

From this we can draw the important conclusion that all plant forms contain the necessary nutrients for sustaining animal organisms. In some plants they appear in a scattered form, in others they are highly concentrated. Among natural foods the most nutritious plant bodies are avocados, bananas, cherimoya, grapes, lemons, mangos, nectarines, oranges, peaches, strawberries, tomatoes, watermelons, and all the other fruits and seeded vegetables. After which comes the roots, herbs, and greens.

Those nutritive constituents that are found in a concentrated state in the fruit of a tree are also found dispersed sparsely in leaves, bark, and branches. A giant animal like the giraffe nourishes itself by feeding on tree leaves. When a small bud of a tree is grafted upon another tree, it shoots forth branches and eventually gives the corresponding fruit. This is a clear indication that a bud contains all the elementary constituents that are essential for the formation of a given fruit.

Now what are those elementary constituents? They are the atoms, which may be regarded as the smallest chemically indivisible particle of an element that can take part in a chemical change, and the molecules, which are the smallest particles of a compound. All edible plants consist of almost the same elements arranged in different proportions to form various compounds. They only differ from one another in form, color, and taste. Thus, clover and sheep are exactly the same. On being introduced into the stomach of a sheep, the molecular structure of clover undergoes a metamorphosis and becomes the sheep. There is a similar correspondence between fruit and humans.

All plant and animal life is nothing but an eternal interchange and circulation of atoms. It is here that the infinite wisdom of Nature asserts itself. We throw into the ground a tiny seed. After a few days it sprouts. Then it shoots forth branches and leaves. In due course it gives fruit. Later that fruit is changed into an ant, a wild sow, or a human which roams about this world for a while and then returns its atoms to the Earth. There, under the vivifying influence of sunlight, those very atoms are revived afresh, new life is breathed into them and they are turned once more into the same plants and animals, to repeat the everlasting cycle of life over and over again. This cycle of life is severely altered by the toxic nature of dead, decomposing, cooked-food humans. They are literally "pushing *down* the daisies."

It is of worthy note that the same principles of nutrition that hold true for animals also hold true for plants. Plants get diseases when there are no longer any elements in the soil to supply them with their nutritional demands. Plants also become subject to diseases when toxins, poisons, and artificial chemicals leach into their root or respiratory structures, filter into their living fluids, and become trapped in their plant fibers.

In order that plant food may give birth to specialized, healthy, and highly-evolved cells, it must not only be complete and living but it must also be active and not dormant. For example, wheatberries and almonds should be sprouted (activated) before consumption. It must be said that humans are not a "sproutarian" species. Sprouts have an affinity for water. When they are ingested, they dehydrate the digestive organs of the body. They may clog the body's sewage system much like cooked food. Sprout consumption should be limited to the winter season.

Experience has shown us that house birds are not satisfied with dry seeds alone. They demand some fresh food as well. The particular variety of those seeds or the fresh food is not important. Perfect nourishment can be obtained by choosing a certain variety of seed or grain and supplementing it with any fresh fruit or soft vegetable.

This fact brings us to the important conclusion that the most perfect food ceases to be perfect after it is dried. Keeping this in mind, it is truly mind-boggling that people regard those substances that come out of ovens, microwaves, toasters, boxes, cans, boiling water, and the jaws of roaring machines as nourishment.

Nevertheless, animal organisms (including natural humans) do not suffer serious harm when they are deprived of fresh foods during the few months of winter. For they make up the deficiency during the bountiful spring and summer, when all Nature comes to life again. Nature has inured them to that mode of life.

Dried seeds, nuts, and legumes are indeed living foodstuffs, but they are in an inert and dormant state. Fortunately, they can easily be aroused, activated, and turned into perfect foods by being soaked in water and kept in cool air for one or two days. Therefore, by the consumption of only sprouted grains the human being has the opportunity to secure perfect nutrition in all seasons of the year and in every corner of the globe.

People go through tremendous expense to publish numerous books to demonstrate the therapeutic properties of individual fruits and vegetables, such as grapefruit, strawberries, garlic, or broccoli. By developing special methods of consuming them, they try to invest those operations with a semblance of scientific progress. In point of fact, all edible varieties of raw fruits and vegetables are perfectly formed nutriments and have essentially the same qualities. No matter what the person's state of health, these nutriments completely satisfy the demands of the organs; they regulate the functions of the organism; they restore lost life.

Cooked food is poison.

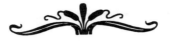

Chapter 35

Cooked-Food Scientists Know Nothing

*"It is notorious, universally so, that the
blackest of falsehoods are ever decked out
in the most brilliant and gorgeous regalia."*
— **Ragnar Redbeard**

In the last chapter you saw that all edible plants consist of the same elements, and that differences in their chemical and physical properties are due to differences in their composition and molecular structure. Unfortunately, scientists have ignored this irrefutable fact and have based their whole science on those few complex compounds they have found in foods. Inebriated by their "discoveries," they have closed their eyes to the most wonderful laboratory of all: Nature. Under the right conditions we can sow a seed so small that it is barely visible to the naked eye and in a few months time reap a majestic plant which fulfills all our alimentary desires.

But scientists don't pay any heed to this. Molecular biology now dominates the thinking of "health-professionals" and, in turn, they have neglected the major effects of nutrition. They proceed unceasingly to burn and destroy living foods. They prepare, in their miserable laboratories, some dead, derivative substances which bear a corrupt resemblance to the original. They then dignify these concoctions with various names and numbers and use them to "repair" the organs of sick people.

By the most inhumane and unnatural means, these scientists search the organs of animals and discover in them various substances, such as proteins, fats, and carbohydrates. They then look for those substances in different foods. Whenever they find something resembling one of them, they regard it as an essential nutrient and recommend that food to all. They never take into account the holistic qualitative and quantitative properties of those foods.

Nutritionists tell people to consume proteins, since "proteins build muscle and strength." But how much should be consumed? Is there a generally agreed upon figure?

Foods in which they manage to find a prominent type of substance are recommended as the source of that given substance. Having found several different substances in grapefruits, they say that grapefruits are rich in those certain elements, as if they contained nothing else. They use the same approach when analyzing all foods — natural or non-natural. As a result of such myopic research, the most harmful foods are represented as fully-balanced nutrients and vice versa.

List in your mind all of the substances which biologists have discovered in the unnatural foods obtained from a cow: milk, yogurt, cheese, butter, sour cream, muscle (beef), liver, heart, etc. Could they detect all those foods in grasses and clover? No way. No one can deny the fact that the raw materials which developed the cow's body are none other than raw plant foods. Except for the difference of one central atom, chlorophyll (plant "blood") is molecularly identical to hemoglobin (human blood). Chlorophyll is centered on magnesium, hemoglobin on iron.

The whole cow is formed entirely of grasses and water. The complete carcass of a carnivore's freshly-killed prey, with its skin, blood, flesh, and bones, has a nutritive value equal to that of grass. But what value does milk and dead cow muscle (steak) have when taken separately? Each of them, even if eaten raw, has an infinitesimal fraction of the value of common grass — as to what remains of those substances after cooking requires no elucidation. Thus the true nutritive value of milk and cow muscle, the foods so worshipped by people, is now exposed. It does not take a genius to judge the real worth of all those milk and meat advertisements that flood the media. We demand that the disseminators of such lies be made aware of the atrocious crimes they commit. The responsibility for the death of millions of people rests squarely on their shoulders.

Now, admittedly, humans are curious creatures, ever anxious to learn new things, to penetrate into Nature's secrets, to broaden the horizons of knowledge. So why don't we let research scientists confine their investigations to the three walls of their laboratory — we are giving them a wall — until the day when they succeed in nurturing a seed to a full-grown, healthy plant with entirely synthetic elements. At that point their wisdom will be equal to that of Nature.

Fortunately, the world is already full of seeds which grow fantastically into magnificent plants and feed the animals of the world. Natural nutrients are free from the slightest defect. No natural substance is redundant; each constituent has its quality and quantity determined by the most accurate calculations. Those who doubt this, doubt the supreme wisdom of Nature; indeed they come into direct conflict with the very principles which give them existence.

New "experts" have stepped into an inviolable realm. They have displaced the best engineer imaginable and now wish to run an organic machine consisting of trillions of cells. Everywhere there are fragments of raw materials scattered among a clanjam-fry of dead materials. As they enter the organism, all are thrown together at random. People enter into a mad frenzy to pluck smoldering ashes off of grills and out of stoves. Everybody chokes their own living machine with whatever they desire. Experiments are made...endless experiments.

Naturally enough, the organic machine begins to malfunction. The more irregularly the machine works, the more do these specialists multiply their efforts. They flail to and fro looking for new methods and new materials. In their whirlwind they trample, destroy, and burn those essential organic compounds found in natural foods.

When they see that their efforts are of no avail and that the machine's condition has gone from bad to worse, they go still further into the city and find completely new substances that have no connection whatsoever to the normal functioning of the machine. For a while one of those new substances stops the machine's overproduction, another slows down certain mechanisms, yet another redirects the operations of some systems. These changes appear as good signs to cooked-food addicts. They leap for joy and raise their arms. They then proceed to search for "stronger," "more effective" substances. Sometimes certain parts of the machine shut down entirely endangering the safety of their neighbors. It is at this point that medical science shows its great dexterity; cooked-food surgeons skillfully remove and cast away those "useless" parts.

It is not surprising that all those efforts end in utter failure. One after another each machine collapses, but the bumbling engineers do not lose hope. They persist in their demented experiments, refusing to recall the real engineer of those machines — Nature — whom they have denied.

The continual comparison of the human body to a machine is not done in a literal sense. Though the analogy is instructive, the human organism is six million times more complicated than any machine ever devised. Its components are so small that most of them are invisible and incomprehensible. A machine has no conscience. Unlike any machine, the human organism is bathed in the life-force which defies description and definition.

So-called "experts" carry out experiments on human beings by the most terrible instruments available, by the most disgusting concoctions imaginable, by ludicrous synthetic preparations, and by all the deadly poisons known to humanity. They publish endless lists of unintelligible substance names and lead people astray with their recommendations. They suggest what they fancy, they say what comes to mind — the whole process is entirely done at random. They fill thousands of books and flood the media with lies. Everything they do is false, everything they say is contradictory. They represent the most harmful substances as exceedingly beneficial, but they forbid the use of that which is essential. In this cacophony of confusion, the experts themselves stand in a maze craze of doubt and indecision, while their audience remains perplexed and mystified. In the meantime, millions of people, having only known a polluted existence, make their early departure from this world. All this is for the sake of addiction.

We appeal to all courageous people throughout the world to come out of their apathetic indifference, if only for the sake of their own and their family's health. Let them join with us so that our united forces may open the eyes of all humanity. In this way we can put an end to the world's present feeding customs and halt all those worthless massacres.

Everybody needs to open their eyes and carefully observe the shocking scams that disgrace all civilization. Due to scientific ignorance, profiteers and speculators have engulfed the whole field of nutrition. The most harmful and grossly adulterated foods are freely advertised as rich sources of vitamins and minerals and are openly marketed to the public. They include: chocolates, muffins, soft drinks, ice creams, frozen yogurts, dried meats, flavored milks, protein powders, and thousands of other items which have been totally deprived of their most vital nutrients and are especially prone to cause illnesses and kill people. The most frightening substances are collected from different factories and bakeries, mixed together, placed in plastic containers, labeled with seemingly scientific names, and sold to the gullible masses at exorbitant prices. The pharmaceutical industry makes so much money that they sometimes pay doctors upwards of a fifty percent commission on pills prescribed by them. One could fill thousands of books on the corruption in just this one industry today. We are not at leisure to even touch that subject here.

It has taken research biologists until the present day to finally notice that some vitamins are not just simple compounds, but elaborate conglomerates of dozens of substances. Gradually, they have noticed that certain vitamins do not show their potency in the absence of others. They have observed that, upon being introduced into the organism, one substance changes into another (e.g., the body converts Beta-carotene into Vitamin A).

The effects of artificial vitamins on the human organism are apparent and contradictory. Inferior, extracted vitamins never penetrate the inner layers of the cellular structure. They may protect the outer layers for time and only from some types of damage. If they are used excessively they may intoxicate the cells. This is precisely what happens when a patient dies immediately after a vitamin injection. How can one possibly represent as "health-giving" a substance which, even in small quantities, may kill a person six minutes after it enters the body? When will doctors abandon such folly and come to their senses? In spite of the multitude of failures, disappointments, and disasters, the medical establishment still persists in its apocalyptic approach. The definition of insanity is: Doing the same things over and over and expecting a different result. Success leaves clues, so does failure. But they refuse to retreat even a single step.

Let us just assume for a moment that all the books written on weight loss, vitamins, minerals, proteins, fats, disease prevention, etc. are true. That would mean that everybody who lives on the planet would be under a necessity to memorize all those books by heart. What would happen to the millions of people who live far from civilization, in the mountains and valleys, in distant villages and hamlets. Must they too familiarize themselves with all the dietary prescriptions laid out by pseudo-intellectuals? Must they die early deaths, in ignorance? In actuality, those who live farthest from civilization live far longer, healthier lives because they are deep within the heart of Nature.

The diets prescribed in thousands of books are not suitable for humanity. All those books which deal with the functions and "benefits" of proteins, fats, carbohydrates, vitamins, and minerals should be silenced. So should all those dangerous publications in which attempts are made to prove that the value of certain foods lies in some particular nutrient contained therein. *How Nature would rejoice if these books were burned in the same fashion in which they recommend our food should be treated.*

At most, future research should be directed towards general experiments which compare certain classes of foods with other classes. For example, studies might be made to ascertain the differences between fruits, vegetables, herbs, sprouts, nuts, legumes, beans, roots, and leaves, if such differences do, in fact, exist.

The only way to free humanity from its present situation is to introduce a radical change in its feeding customs and living conditions. These habits must be harmonized to blend the correct system of nutrition with the biological goals of humankind. Every single one of the items people consume should be a complete and perfect food.

It is possible to lead humanity along the correct path, because Nature constantly culls out those individuals unfit for reproduction. Masses of cooked humanity are headed towards genetic dead-ends which will manifest themselves in sooner or later generations. We must remember that Nature's plans operate not just during a lifetime: its grand designs span generations, naye thousands of generations. Humanity's concept of time is arbitrary and has nothing to do with a bird's or a tree's concept of time. So, eventually, it is possible to succeed as long as the scientific facts are available to anyone.

We desire to create such conditions as will make it feasible for rich and poor, great and small, learned and simple people alike to lead healthy lives without being under the threat of any disease or debilitation. Their choice of foods will be determined by their alimentary instinct, their entire bodies will be nourished simply by following their inner commands.

When people set out on any endeavor they should have a clear prevision of their goal. Unfortunately, research scientists and biologists have never enunciated their final objective — so we will tell them. They are trying to find out what sort of substances the human body needs in order to lead a healthy life. They wish to ascertain the proper functions of each vitamin, mineral, enzyme, protein, fat, and carbohydrate in the human organism.

Through their endless work and toil, they have finally ascertained that a certain vitamin enlivens the muscles, a certain mineral strengthens the teeth, a certain enzyme aids in the digestion of fiber, etc. But instead of subjecting themselves to all that trouble, would it not be better if they observed the way in which Nature works? Why don't they ask the gorillas what variety of proteins or protein powders they consume to accumulate their enormous muscular body which gives them the ability to individually bench press over four-thousand pounds?

Research scientists are educated, but they are completely devoid of any instinct, as are all "civilized" and "cultured" peoples. They would rather do anything than to give up their beloved bread. Is eating raw wheat too "primitive" for them? *Or is it just too natural?* They never allow us to forget that lifeless starches and sugars have their "benefits." They fill the stomach, and alleviate any hunger. All those missing nutrients can of

course be supplemented by such "marvelous" scientific resources as artificial vitamins, protein drinks, and amino acid
pills.

If the facts about nutrition were to get out, what would
happen to all their hospitals, "health" officials, pharmacies, and
multi-level marketing vitamin companies? How could they abandon all those "achievements" and their pasta too? Such a step
cannot even be fathomed by an indoctrinated mind. To those
brainwashed scientists, it matters very little that millions of
people spend their lives engaging in worthless unnatural activities
and then die of heart disease, cancer, or diabetes. Sooner or later
all people must die anyway, so why not party and pollute and
then leave this world in a bang? What is the use in having a
plethora of children and living to the age of one hundred and
sixty in a world which is overcrowded? Most pseudo-intellectuals
have this attitude in mind. Indeed, most human beings, blinded
as they are by addictions, think in this way. To this we do solemnly
declare to the whole world: Bread is the most addictive substance
on the planet. We attack those religions which believe that a tiny
bread wafer is the body of their god and cooked grapes are the
blood. All wheat and grapes must be consumed in their raw,
living state.

Instead of analyzing outdated, unnatural ideas, scientists
should first empty their minds of all preconceptions and then
make observations. By using inductive logic one could generalize
from these observations about particular cases. In this way one
would finally arrive at the most fundamental and comprehensive
Laws of Nature. Once cooked-food scientists realize that they
know basically nothing, then they will finally have learned
something.

Cooked food is poison.

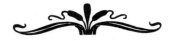

Chapter 36

Detoxification

"Nature never did betray the heart that loved her."
— **William Wordsworth**

During the initial period of raw-eating, cooked-foodists experience various discomforts, which give thoughtless people the false impression that natural foods exhaust the body and impair health. This misconception is the most striking proof of humanity's short-sightedness. The mere idea that natural nutrition may be followed by unnatural and harmful results is a most absurd notion which must be stricken from the minds of everyone once and for all.

Fifty to sixty kilograms of a person weighing one hundred kilograms belongs to a false body which immediately begins to dissolve on a raw-food diet. At that point, diseased cells, fat excretions, dead water, and other poisons rush into the blood stream to be purged from the system. The body makes use of all its eliminative organs: the skin, bowels, mouth, sinuses, and urine in order to rid itself of those vile toxins.

On observing foreign substances in the feces or urine, short-sighted people believe they are formed from natural nutriments. Actually, they come from the disgusting, undigested cooked foods that make up the false body — which is gradually wasting away. The transition to raw-foodism must not be controlled by the usual, milquetoast criteria of medical science; people must submit whole-heartedly to Nature's First Law. The results of raw-foodism take months, sometimes years (if someone lived an abominable life-style); they must be awaited with strength, patience, and perseverance.

During the detoxification process, symptoms of intestinal discomfort, gas, headaches, light-headedness, nausea, rashes, etc. may appear. In certain cases the urine may become cloudy. The feet may swell, sores may appear on the body, and there may be dryness and itching on the scalp and skin. All these are processes of detoxification and healing; the good pushing out the bad. No one should succumb to their feelings of "hunger" and return to those "nutritious" and "well-balanced" meals of the past. Should one be foolish enough to do so, these cleansing symptoms immediately disappear, but, of course, to the detriment of one's health. The false body will then heave a sigh of relief and, laughing at the stupidity of the true body, will begin to grow once again with a new lease on life.

Your mind will play tricks on you as negative impulses and unnatural desires are also purged from the system. Embrace those experiences, and get past them. Hold tenaciously to your goal and never, ever, lose hope in the healing power of Nature. Strengthening the subconscious undomesticates.

Detoxification symptoms vary in occurrence and severity from one individual to another, they typically follow cyclical patterns. They may be entirely absent in some people. As a rule, they are apt to be severe in elderly and obese people, mild in young people, and completely absent in newborn children. In a fat person, the false body has so suffocated and emaciated the true body under the pressure of heavy weight, that little is left but skin and bones.

As a rule, pets tend to experience mild detoxification symptoms when they are fed a raw diet.

In the initial period of raw-eating an individual's weight will be reduced so much that those who do not comprehend its true nature will begin to criticize and debase that individual. What they see is merely an apparent picture of what is taking place. In the body of a raw-foodist the true body has, in fact, begun to gain weight. After the false body is completely crushed the raw-foodist will continue to gain until an ideal body weight is attained. In a very thin person the increase in the weight of the true body will counterbalance the loss suffered by the false body, so that there will be an overall net gain in weight.

This growth of the true body is particularly fast in ashen, emaciated, and weak children. People must not expect raw children to be as chubby-faced and pudgy-legged as their cooked peers, for obesity is the sign of the false body. Children fed exclusively raw foods will be lean, muscular, and powerful. It is through sheer ignorance that simple-minded, cooked-food parents rejoice at the plumpness of their children.

When we became raw-eaters, an extensive process of purification commenced in our bodies. We experienced symptoms of drowsiness, mouth sores, bad breath, intestinal purging, and a few other minor ailments. During the whole detoxification period we exercised more and more extensively by taking long walks in Nature; walking creates wisdom.

We discovered that whenever any of us ate any cooked food, we would gain 2 to 3 kilograms because the cooked food would act as a plug in the body's sewage system. It may even be good, in an enlightened sense, for a new raw-foodist to revert to past cooked habits after a long period of abstinence from cooked food. By comparing the two systems of nutrition, s/he becomes all the more convinced that the raw path is indeed the right one.

In contravention of these minor problems, we acquired enormous advantages. The following are some of the benefits of raw-foodism we have experienced:
- Elimination of pollen and animal allergies.
- Improved eyesight.
- Quick and strong growth of hair and fingernails.
- Increased resistance to cold and hot weather.
- Faster reflexes.
- Invulnerability to sunburn and a better tan.
- Increased endurance and energy.
- Better sense of smell and hearing.
- The ability to breathe deeper and hold our breath longer.
- Fresher breath and a decreased body odor.
- Only 4 to 6 hours of sleep required each night.
- The ability to fast with no adverse effects.
- Clearer, more logical thinking.
- Greater concentration, memory, and mental focus.

- Superior attitude towards life, Nature, and the order of things.
- A closer relationship with natural forces.
- Increased confidence.
- Decreased stress.
- Increased affinity for innate desires.
- Increased individualism.
- Increased sexual energy.
- Controlled temper.

The list goes on and on...
Cooked food is poison.

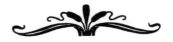

Chapter 37

Infectious Diseases

"The specific disease doctrine is the grand
refuge of weak, uncultured, unstable minds, such as
now rule the medical profession. There are no specific
diseases; there are specific disease conditions."
— **Florence Nightingale**

The claims that the danger of infectious diseases is steadily on the decline are fallacious. Because of cooked-eating human cells have gradually lost their power of resistance to microbes and, what is worse, they continue losing that power from generation to generation.

There are a number of infections particular to Homo sapiens (anthroponoses) that do not, in fact, occur in animals, including the primates. Scientists either do not succeed in inducing experimental examples of those infections in them or else they manage to obtain a very remote resemblance of only a few of them (typhoid, cholera, malaria, meningococcal meningitis, influenza, measles, jaundice, diphtheria, scarlet fever, pneumonia, rheumatism, sepsis, gonorrhea, furunculosis, appendicitis, etc.).

The zoonoses and ornithonoses (animal and bird diseases) that occur in human beings, such as hydrophobia, encephalitis, brucellosis (Malta fever), psittacosis, smallpox, plague, tularemia, anthrax, trichinosis, and others have, as a rule, their special symptoms that are peculiar to humans, whereas in animals sometimes they show only very remote reproductions of those symptoms.

It thus appears that not only do all animals, including humanity's closest relatives, the apes, not contract specific human infections, but they are not even responsive to the deliberate attempts of research scientists to infect them with those diseases for experimental purposes. In contrast, there exist bacteria that are particular to animals and birds, but do not adversely affect them, even though they are continuously present in their organs. On being transmitted to humans, however, those very bacteria multiply in a most terrible and disastrous manner. We must add to this the fact that wild animals are immune from all chronic diseases.

What is the reason for this striking contrast? The difference lies first and foremost in the nutritional habits of "civilized" humanity. No free-born animal ever tampers with its food. Free-living animals do not "improve" their food. They do not eat any unnatural or artificial meals. They keep their tissues pure and healthy. As a result, they do not know disease — infectious or otherwise. They know only full, unrelenting life — and death.

The fight against infectious diseases proceeds from a completely mistaken standpoint. The decline in the death-rate from infectious diseases has been achieved not by strengthening the resistance of the body, but by mitigating the external conditions that spread infections. In course of time humanity's power of resistance has been so weakened that if we removed the amenities provided by modern housing, centralized water-supply systems, urban sanitation, isolation of patients and so forth, and returned to the conditions prevailing two hundred years ago, the human race would be annihilated through various epidemic diseases within a few years.

But even with improved sanitation, auto-infections develop quickly and become an inevitable disaster for all cooked-eating humanity. Taking advantage of the weak cells spread throughout the false body, harmless micro-organisms become quite harmful. Contemporary data indicates that bacteria may undergo a metamorphosis. That is, pathogenic bacteria may be produced from so-called non-pathogenic bacteria. Thus, the bacilli of typhoid, paratyphoid, and dysentery may originate from the intestinal bacilli; the real bacilli of diphtheria may develop from benign bacilli. Such metamorphoses may take place in all varieties of cocci, in anaerobes, in the bacilli of different plagues, tuberculosis, and in other micro-organisms.

In a great many infectious diseases the bacterial origin for the infection is absent. Generally speaking, every infectious disease makes its first appearance in the delicate organism of some weakly cooked-foodist and is thence transmitted to other people. In reality, every such organism is a dangerous factory for the propagation and dissemination of pathogenic bacteria. Such a factory is not to be found among raw-foodists. So the world of raw-foodists will be forever free from all infectious diseases.

The main regions of the body where auto-infections develop are: the throat, the tonsils, the vermiform appendix, the large intestine, the conjunctiva, the bronchial tubes, and the urinary passages. These are the eliminative organs, which become taxed and fatigued by cooked food. They eventually clog up and become breeding grounds for bacteria.

In regard to the etiology of infectious diseases you must abandon the notions conceived by Kircher, Ehrlich, and Pasteur on the "pathogenic" nature of micro-organisms. In the full sense of the word it is not the bacteria themselves that are pathogenic, but those physiological environments that exist in the given organism at that particular moment. These disturbances are organically connected with the disturbances in particles ingested by the organism. There are no special "pathogenic" microbes in Nature; there are, however, no end to the factors that promote susceptibility in a normally resistant subject.

We can draw only one logical conclusion from all this. The real cause of infectious diseases is not the microbe, but the impaired condition of the normal biological processes of the organism. In the past century, Professor Antoine Bechamp showed that microzymes (the smallest unit of life) remained normal under compatible conditions, but developed into bacteria and parasites when presented with putrefied or fermented food. Even the notorious Louis Pasteur admitted on his deathbed that "the microbe is nothing, the terrain is everything." Pasteur, who suffered from severe, cooked-food paralysis for most of the latter half of his life, was never able to elaborate on his admission because he died of cellular starvation.

The belief that humans, the prodigal product of millions of years of animal evolution, remain defenseless against some microscopic germ that sneaks into the body, multiplies, and destroys everything, is totally ridiculous, and must be abolished. Only the ingestion of unnatural substances lowers the body's natural defenses.

Germs (prokaryotic bacteria) have always existed, they still exist, and they will exist forever. To combat disease by attempting to destroy germs is sheer folly. Germs are found everywhere. Through multifarious pathways, these tiny microbes continually enter and exit our bodies. They are the earliest successful organisms to appear on the planet. They lived and evolved on Earth all alone for two billion years before the emergence of plant and animal life. Most germs serve one vital function: they change organic matter into inorganic matter. Wherever there is decay, germs are there to purify. Countless different types of these germs exist in symbiotic relationships with the human organism.

Additionally, all the germ principles hold true for so-called "viruses" as well. However, the virus theory is on even less stable ground than the germ theory. There is not one bit of scientific evidence that proves that viruses are even alive! Unlike all other living creatures they do not ingest nutrients, eliminate waste, move independently, or maintain any kind of internal homeostatic balance. Viruses may well be DNA lifeboats (they rescue DNA from certain destruction within poisoned, emaciated, dying cells) or they may be the nucleic debris of dead, ruptured cells being recycled back into living cells. This would explain why viruses tend to increase in number as the cells in the body die in greater numbers (such as during sickness).

A prime example of the completely ludicrous virus theory is the HIV/AIDS (Human Immune-deficiency Virus/Acquired Immune Deficiency Syndrome) hypothesis formed by present day biologists and scientists. The entire HIV and AIDS scare is a total fraud from top to bottom. It is fueled by money and sexual repression. In fact, it can be proven that AIDS is not an infectious disease at all. AIDS deaths are nothing more than severe cases of total immune system breakdown caused by autointoxication, accompanied by the benign HIV.

For the sake of argument, let us assume that viruses do, in fact, exist. Under current medical terminology, HIV fits the category of a retrovirus. According to Dr. Peter Duesberg, a molecular biologist at the University of California at Berkeley and the "discoverer" of retroviruses, HIV is infectious, but extremely difficult to transmit. Dr. Duesberg convincingly argues that the presence of HIV in a human host simply indicates that a person has engaged in acts the AIDS Establishment terms "high-risk behavior" which include: intravenous drug use, blood exchange, and/or unprotected sex with multiple partners (most prevalent in male homosexuals). Even high-risk behavior does not always pass the virus from one person to another. HIV does not, by any means, indicate that an AIDS case is inevitable. In fact, only 1.5% of people that have tested positive for HIV are diagnosed with AIDS in any given year.

Upon infection, HIV spreads extremely mildly. It actively infects, at most, one in ten-thousand T-cells (these cells are responsible for cellular and long-term immune reactions). Every two days the body regenerates T-cells at a rate of 5%, or 500 times faster than the virus can actively infect them. According to Dr. Duesberg, the structure of HIV is a very simple mechanism and its "life" cycle is such that it can only go around the clock one time. It infects a cell from the inside out, the human organism develops HIV antibodies, and the virus is purged out of the body in a very short time. When someone tests positive for HIV, they are actually only testing positive for the presence of HIV antibodies; the virus is gone. The idea that it can lie dormant in a human host for one, five, ten, or twenty years (the AIDS Establishment keeps extending it) and then suddenly explode and destroy the organism is totally ridiculous. This is not at all the way in which a simple virus works. They work fast, or never.

Additionally, the propaganda propounded upon the masses that a major epidemic exists is prima facie preposterous. In fact, more people die every year from sleeping pill overdoses than from AIDS. The high-risk groups for AIDS have not changed in fifteen years. No epidemic can be that selective. If HIV transmitted easily it would have spread randomly into the population. It has not; AIDS has not. The predictions continue to fall. In the

United Kingdom, 17,000 deaths had been predicted for 1992. This was slashed to 5,000.

The prediction numbers have gotten so low that the AIDS definition has to be expanded to keep the numbers justified (which they never are). Every year there is a new HIV "strain," more diseases, a longer latency period, mycoplasmic cofactors, etc.

HIV was announced as the cause of AIDS in 1984 by the United States Secretary of Health under extremely unscientific medical standards. It was not published in a single medical journal before the announcement. To say that AIDS is definitely caused by HIV is, even if it were true, an extreme over-simplification. AIDS has multiple manifestations and the Establishment has now taken at least 25 known diseases that, when accompanied by HIV, indicates an AIDS case. No longer is the cause of death pneumonia, tuberculosis, or Kaposi's sarcoma (a rare cancer), but the HIV virus. Really, they juggle one mistaken cause of death for another more outlandish one.

As mentioned, AIDS is caused by autointoxication. As its name suggests, Acquired Immune Deficiency Syndrome, develops over time until the body, through massive poisoning, begins to fail. For cases in which the patients are male homosexuals and intravenous drug users, this poisoning stems from non-infectious agents such as malnutrition (cooked food) and/or daily consumption of recreational drugs, sometimes for years at a time. In the hard-core drug and homosexual communities, these drugs include: cocaine, heroin, alcohol, cooked marijuana, ethyl chloride, amyl nitrates ("poppers"), as well as designer drugs such as Ecstasy, Special K, and MDA. Just one of these poisonous drugs wreaks havoc upon the body, let alone six or seven of these drugs taken at once for extended periods of time. For example, poppers, a type of nitrate inhalant which facilitates anal sex, are known to combine with synthetic antibiotics, such as penicillin and tetracycline, in the laboratory to form carcinogens; this is the leading hypothesis for the cause of Kaposi's sarcoma. It is Kaposi's sarcoma, not a virus, which causes the purple lesions on the skin of AIDS patients.

Any sensible person can clearly see that nothing is more immuno-suppressive than the prolonged consumption of unnatural substances. The media portrays many AIDS patients as poor, unfortunate people who die because they are indiscriminately stricken with a "deadly" virus. Once again, it is the "unwillingness to accept the responsibility for one's own actions" principle in action.

For hemophiliacs and others who contract HIV through blood transfusions, it must be said that blood transfusions are themselves extremely immuno-suppressive, dangerous, and unnatural. Nature did not design the human organism to carry the blood of another human. It is no surprise that such a procedure may eventually kill a person because of the foreign blood, upon injection, spreads to every capillary in the body. It is also interesting to note that hemophiliacs that are HIV positive and those that are HIV negative have exactly the same incidence of disease.

Keeping all this in mind, we see that the AIDS Establishment, in their "infinite wisdom," have chosen to ignore the obvious and fight AIDS with its "wonder drug," AZT (now euphemized under the name of Retrovir). AZT, which theoretically destroys HIV, actually terminates DNA synthesis. DNA is the basis for all life on the planet. It is, in fact, very difficult to determine if a patient is dying of AIDS or by the toxic effects of the drug. AZT is one of the most potent poisons ever developed. No one has ever lived more than three years while taking AZT.

The AIDS Establishment will continue to fail and lie, ad infinitum. Even if viruses do exist, no drug could penetrate into the cellular chemistry and wipe out one infinitely small agent without destroying everything in its path. In fact, Dr. Duesberg compares the curative process of AZT to "hunting rabbits with the Neutron bomb; sure you will kill the rabbits, but you will destroy the entire forest in the process."

Short-sighted opponents of Dr. Duesberg believe that his ideas have been outdated. Common sense and logic *cannot be* outdated. Due to the "Great International Money Tower" and political pressure, it has been extremely difficult for Dr. Duesberg and others with alternative hypotheses to get their ideas into the mainstream public, which has been brainwashed with the stagnant, "conventional wisdom" of the time. Friedrich Nietzsche once said, "What everybody believes, is never true." *When true geniuses emerge, it is easy to spot them; all the idiots form an alliance against them.*

It has occurred time and time again throughout the course of history that the ideas of true geniuses and innovators go through three stages. First, the new idea is immediately scorned. Second, it is violently opposed. Finally, when it is proven to be true, it is accepted and practiced as the norm.

It happened to Nicolaus Copernicus, whose idea of a heliocentric solar system challenged the geocentric cosmology that had been dogmatically accepted since the time of Aristotle. The work that he did is traditionally considered the inauguration of the scientific revolution.

It happened to Galileo Galilei, whose discoveries conflicted so greatly with the Roman Catholic Church, that he was taken to Rome and forced to abjure, on his knees, the views he had expressed in his book. Ever since, Galileo has been portrayed as a victim of a repressive church and a martyr in the cause of freedom of thought.

And now it is happening to Dr. Duesberg. His research grant was not renewed when he came forward with his hypothesis that challenged the AIDS Money Establishment. When they are finally willing to accept the fact that Dr. Duesberg's hypothesis is correct, they will realize that many lives that could have been saved, were not; the very hallmark of a poorly founded hypotheses.

And, inevitably, it will happen with this book, with our exposing of the Raw-food/Cooked-food Truth.

As a result of turning a blind eye to the real causes of diseases, humanity's organic power of resistance has been gradually reduced to such an extent that human beings no longer await for infection to come from without, but succumb to the bacteria swarming inside their bodies. For in the human organism those very bacteria that are unable to do any harm to the fiercest of animals come face to face with weak, worthless, inactive cells formed from cooked animal muscles, processed sugar, bread, and pasteurized cow's milk. It is no wonder, then, that they simply fall upon those cells and devour them avidly. Sensible people should cleanse their bodies of every single one of those useless cells, after which no microbe will dare approach the youthful, robust, and strong cells that will have come into existence from noble fruits, vegetables, and herbs.

The role of antibiotics as therapeutic agents is temporary and deceptive. People are gradually becoming disappointed with them. Neutralizing the effects of bacterial activity for a short spell of time, they weaken the cells and clear the way for stronger infections later on.

Many hospital patients die every day from the adverse effects of antibiotics. For example, as a result of a deficiency of natural nutrition some patients suffer from an irregular, persistent fever caused by auto-infection and self-poisoning. Their temperatures usually fluctuate between 37.5 and 38 degrees Celsius (99.5 and 100.5 degrees Fahrenheit). Entrusted to the most eminent "specialists," these patients, through indiscriminate experimentation with synthetic antibiotics, have their temperatures raised to 40 to 41 degrees Celsius (104 to 106 degrees Fahrenheit). They are literally cooked. Their hearts and kidneys unwittingly degenerated, they are finally killed without ever receiving the proper diagnosis.

Every day doctors draw enormous quantities of blood. These samples are subjected to various laboratory tests or injected into dozens of rats. Doctors then pretend that by multiplying the bacteria they might identify the actual organism which was responsible for the disease. They never can determine this in their clinical examinations. The higher the temperature of the patient goes, the larger the doses of antibiotics that are administered and the more diverse are the varieties of those poisons.

Fortunate patients that get out of the hospital in time and entrust their health to natural nutrition have remarkable recoveries. Of course, the doctors label these cases as "spontaneous remission" and pay no heed to the true cure: Raw-foodism. Unfortunately, many patients revert to their old cooked-eating habits and fall victim to disease once again. Remember, it is a

most errant notion to consider raw plant food as only a therapeutic means. Raw-foodism is the only way to live naturally and
normally.

Cooked food is poison.

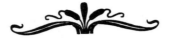

Chapter 38

Our Experience With Raw-Foodism

"I deny all things! I question all things!"
— Ragnar Redbeard

As we have demonstrated, the true body lives on raw food exclusively. All the cooked foods and debased drinks consumed in the world are aimlessly lost. The money spent on them is frivolously wasted. At first sight this statement may seem unbelievable, but it is the simple truth, provable by observation, experiment, and/or personal experience.

In the beginning we thought that we would have to increase the intake of raw nutrition in the same proportion as we reduced the consumption of cooked food. We soon realized we were mistaken. In the initial period of raw-eating, our bodies demanded massive amounts of natural foods in order to restore the persistent losses suffered by the body and to reconstruct the organs by reinforcing them with fresh legions of active cells. Each of us would typically drink a liter of vegetable juice daily along with up to twenty pieces of fruit. As time passed, the demand for large quantities steadily decreased until now we do not eat much at all, perhaps five to ten pieces of fruit each day (mostly just for leisure) while maintaining our ideal weight.

Cooked-foodists are quick to state that raw-eating would limit their food choices. They love unnatural diversity so much. It must be said that raw plant foods are not limited to those seen in western supermarkets. In reality, there are so many types of fruits and vegetables on this planet, that one could try a new one everyday for a hundred years and still not even come close to tasting them all. We have come to enjoy a myriad of new fruits and vegetables which have provided us with sensations and tastes we never before thought imaginable.

It has become clear to us that raw fruits and vegetables are extremely concentrated, high-quality nutriments: a very small quantity of them fully satisfies the needs of the human organism. Breatharianism is no fairy tale. In areas where the life-force is slower, such as the desert and the mountains, people can subsist for months at a time on basically no food at all.

Cooked-foodists can gorge themselves on platefuls of cooked meals, because they contain little nourishment. Herbivorous animals, in their turn, consume huge quantities of vegetation, not because that food is low in nutritional value, but because their digestive organs can only liberate a certain amount of nutrients from the cellulitic fiber. It is the nutrient juice in the fiber of the plant that nourishes the organism. Those animals empty their bowels of roughage several times a day, whereas a natural human experiences only one motion a day.

For a raw-foodist, excessive flatulence, the presence of undigested plant remains in the feces, and the demand to defecate more than once a day are signs of purging or overeating.

Our experiments show that once a false body has been called into existence, partial dietary restrictions are not able to check its development. Even a ten percent degeneration in the quality of ingested food is enough to keep it alive. A sensible person should beware of providing that abomination with even a single cooked grain of nourishment.

The cells of the false body do not retreat with ease. They lie in ambush, half-dead, and dormant, but still expectant. As soon as a piece of degenerated food reaches these cells they revive and multiply.

All weight control should be directed entirely by natural nutrition. People who suggest that being slim is not good for your health are, in effect, recommending that you nurture and nourish dozens of kilograms of sick and parasitic cells in order to maintain the plumpness of the body. Simultaneously with the killing of the false body, natural nutrition will slowly but surely increase the weight of the true body to its ideal proportions. We have experienced this first-hand.

After getting rid of those useless masses of tissue, people who had formerly loaded their bodies with fifty to sixty kilograms of diseased cells and could not climb a step unaided, are able to hike mountains with ease. People should never worry about the rapid loss of weight associated with natural nutrition; they should embrace it, as we have. Intelligent people should not tolerate any quantity of useless flesh on their body. Everybody must finally realize that by introducing even a single morsel of cooked food into the organism, the false body gains nourishment.

It may be said that Truth is the highest virtue, but we have found that living truthfully is higher still.

Cooked food is a callous executioner.

Cooked food is a remorseless enemy.

Cooked food sustains all diseases — known and unknown.

Cooked food is a mad distemper that strikes down both beggar and queen.

Cooked food is poison.

Chapter 39

Summaries

"There are some Truths which are so obvious that for that very reason they are not recognized by ordinary people."
— Nature's First Law

As you have seen, diseases are brought into being by the dissipation of the integral raw materials intended for the human organism. Therefore health can only be recovered if the integrity of those materials is restored. So then we must ask: what is the basis of medical science's activity? What is it that doctors do perform? They make vain attempts to restore that integrity by means of degenerate foods, artificial hormones, synthetic vitamins, and a multitude of poisonous concoctions. At the same time, they remove and discard whole glands and organs that become irreparably damaged and incapacitated as a result of ingesting cooked, dead, and denatured foods and beverages.

All of humankind lives in a state of terrible ignorance. Addicts believe that the consumption of cooked food is something natural, while nourishment by the Laws of Nature is an experiment, and a dangerous experiment at that! In reality, people have unwittingly destroyed the perfect balance developed by Nature. For countless millennia people have been performing asinine experiments by cooking, pickling, and fermenting food. They seek to find a new balance — their own balance. The immediate results of those experiments are the massive pollutants and the numerous diseases that prevail in the world today.

Whenever the question of raw-foodism comes up for discussion, people look at us incredulously and ask: "How can you survive on just raw food?" One cannot find a more absurd utterance in the world. But unfortunately, cooked-food addiction has so blinded humankind that it is, in fact, the usual response of the vast majority of people. Those who lack the necessary experience are in no position to realize how rich and nutritious raw fruits and vegetables are and how little a quantity of these foods is required to satisfy daily needs.

When we invite people to adopt a raw-food diet, we do not propose a new experiment. We simply urge them to put an end to the ludicrous experiments which are always in progress and to return to the natural mode of living. Therefore, anyone who reads these words must not wait for others to carry out that "new experiment" and then wait to be informed of the result. The herd is plundering into the abyss. *There is no safety in numbers.* Anybody with even the least bit of common sense must stop those dangerous experiments and return to the normal way of life. You must return to the natural order.

All those human experiments, the sacred products of human research, have yielded the pills and powders that scientists wish to feed the world. Compare these to beets, celery, and plums which are the sacred products of Nature's laboratory. You make the choice between the two. All cooked foods are artificial substances deprived of their natural qualities. Cooked food is just as bad as those widely-marketed vitamin tablets and freeze-dried food extracts.

Homo sapien has at its disposal the most wholesome and concentrated foods that, having filtered through the leaves and stalks, the trunks and branches of those plants, have come together in their fruits, seeded vegetables (botanical fruits), and nuts. Those edibles have been especially evolved for nourishing the human organism.

The time has come for scientists to admit that they have deviated from the correct path and are conducting their research in entirely erroneous directions. Moreover, they must admit that it is not possible to compensate the losses in natural, raw foods by artificial preparations. They must admit that poisons have no capacity to restore tissue degeneration; the glands and organs of the body are inseparable parts of the human organism that must never be mutilated or removed.

We are showing people a very simple and easy method for relieving the human body from all diseases effectively and conclusively. Diseased and useless cells are destroyed by cutting off the supply of unnatural food. In the stead of that purged dross are the healthy and specialized cells which are produced from natural nutrients. In order to be fully convinced of the validity of our arguments, all one needs do is try eating raw for a few months.

What should be the goal of doctors and biologists, if not the freeing of humankind from disease? Raw-eating is the way to reach that goal. They must declare up front whether they even wish to see a world free from disease. If they can prove that their own calculations are more accurate than the calculations made by Nature and that raw-foodists throughout the world succumb to illnesses instead of recovering their health, we shall immediately cease our efforts, recall all our books, and forever hold our peace. Otherwise, they must put an end to their insidious activities or else declare that they wish only to make money by perpetuating fear, addiction, and insane experiments.

Henceforth, the preparation and recommendation of cooked, dead, and denatured foods will be regarded as crimes against humanity and Nature. Treatments by means of poisons are the alchemy of the present age. People once believed, that by methods of chemistry, lead could be turned into gold. People now believe that by means of chemistry humanity is soon to discover a panacea or an elixir of longevity. We state unequivocally that raw-foodism is the only panacea. *Raw-eating is the Fountain of Youth.*

Wise doctors should immediately stop their bizarre recommendations and invite people to submit to the ordinance of Nature. The hands of the doctors who have a spark of conscience left in their hearts should tremble on writing down the names of poisonous substances and artificial vitamins. Their lips should quiver on pronouncing the names of cooked foods. These operations are tantamount to the passing of a death sentence. Let this be realized by all parents as well.

We consider the recommendation of "chicken soup for the soul," or scrambled egg whites for "strength," or stewed bananas for children a criminal act. This is no slanderous accusation. We do not falsify the facts when we state that all superstitions and medical experiments are really voodoo. Instead of cleansing the blood vessels of heart patients by natural nutrition, doctors choose to widen the blood vessels by irritating poisons. They stimulate the heart by "lashes of the whip" and weaken the patient even more. Such operations are no more advanced than old-fashioned blood-letting. They are deceit and trickery.

Surely we are not guilty of immodesty when, relying on our personal experience and experimentation, we carry out painstaking investigations and then declare that scientists are guilty of pure ignorance when they burn thousands of natural elements, subject the cells to extreme degeneration, and then waste innumerable monetary resources in vain attempts to return to those cells all their lost mechanisms and functions by the discovery of a single artificial substance.

Every scientist understands the complexity of the human organism. A kernel of corn has precisely the same type of complex structure. When it sprouts, it becomes an active and thriving body that lives and breathes. The thousands of substances that are indispensable for the regular operation of all the body's components are precisely calculated. When the living maize is transformed into corn chips, all the substances in it are destroyed, save a few ashes. Imagining those ashes to be real nourishment, well-meaning parents give them to their child, but are afraid to give the child that living corncob.

All the cooked foods in the world, which short-sighted people regard as essential nourishment are nothing but motley heaps of odoriferous and highly-seasoned ashes. The isolated vitamins and corrosive salts discovered in them by biologists are unnatural, lifeless substances. As soon as the living plant cell is cooked, it stops being nourishment and becomes something artificial. When parents give their little baby its first bottle of pasteurized cow's milk, a slice of bread, or some heat-processed baby formula, they begin to perform the most ruthless abuses and inhuman experiments on their child.

Perhaps some people do not like our tone of writing. In their opinion our expressions should preferably be more scientific (adorned with Greek and Latin terminology unintelligible to most people), more conciliatory (milquetoast), more serious (hypocritical), more compromising (unscrupulous), more courteous (filled with lies), more tactful (cowardly). We are driven by forces seeded in our blood. We are decisive and bold. We are accurate and succinct. We hold nothing back and get right to the point. That is how we shall be, even if we find the whole world against us. We are confident that we shall be supported by all sensible people and vindicated by future generations.

The basic error of medical science lies in its deplorable short-sightedness. In this world, it is now possible to arbitrarily fill a group of people with some elementary bits of knowledge, fanciful conjectures, hypothetical assumptions, and contradictory theories, and then grant them complete freedom to toy with the lives of their fellow human beings by means of thousands of poisons, torturous instruments, and arbitrary living regimens. Suppose for a moment that all the medical books and encyclopedias in the world are correct. In order to memorize them a cooked doctor would need twenty lifetimes. Even then s/he would not be able to comprehend one one-thousandth of the innumerable processes operating in the human organism. *People must finally realize that nearly all books ever written are, directly or indirectly, cookbooks.*

If a patient with a chronic disease were to consult a hundred doctors, s/he would receive a hundred different recommendations and prescriptions. For doctors merely perform experiments, and most culpable experiments at that.

In essence, it is the forces of Nature that heal even in spite of the dangerous measures adopted by doctors.

A raw-foods doctor approaches the question of illness from a completely different standpoint. S/he will question patients on their manner of living and on any infringements made upon the Laws of Nature. If such infringements have taken place, the course of treatment may involve sun/air-bathing, fasting, fresh chlorophyll-rich juice, high-water-content fruits, exercise, deep breathing, etc. depending on the doctor's diagnosis. There are no diseases with unknown causes.

Doctors are guilty of the most abominable crimes, even though they do almost everything unintentionally. Now in order that doctors may not repeat the same offense against other people, we must bring an understanding of raw-foodism home to them.

The whole responsibility for repeatedly misguiding the world rests upon the leading specialists: funded research scientists and professors of medicine. Ordinary doctors are really not to be wholly blamed, because they simply put into practice what they have been taught by their professors.

The best minds to date have struggled with the concept of raw-foodism, not because Nature is obscure, but simply because humans find it difficult to outgrow established ways of looking at the world. The time has come when parents and scholars must choose one of the two paths open to them. Either they must accept the infallibility of Nature, embrace its supreme wisdom, and free humanity from its sufferings at once or they must ignore the Laws of Nature and, relying on their own judgment, deem the artificial as superior to the natural.

If they choose to persist in their pernicious experiments the results will be catastrophic. What will be the result if the present state of affairs continues for a few more generations? Massive disease, unnecessary famines, severe pollution, animal mutilation, enslavement, and slaughter, entire populations exhibiting extreme unnatural behaviors — all these will inevitably follow.

Though we strongly attack the present system of healing, we also experience a deep feeling of pity for people, because they have been unknowingly committing unnatural crimes against themselves, their families, and against all of the living world. After reading these lines, those who persist in their errors will be condemned.

Those who turn a deaf ear to these manifest truths today, will not be able to shake off their responsibility tomorrow. When those children of the world mature and find themselves steeped in addictions and living in poor health, they will call into account all teachers and leaders, as well as their own parents and relatives once they discover the facts about nutrition. They will rightly want to know why they were never warned. They will wonder at the crass indifference of their peers.

Do people still think that their wisdom is greater than the wisdom of Nature? If they do not think so, they must put an immediate stop to the destruction of natural foods. This is the absolute command of Nature, which does not allow any compromise. It is the command of that Nature which controls the planet's oceans, atmosphere, jungles, forests, rivers, and lakes by the most perfect laws and ordinances. It is the same Nature that has baffled the human mind for thousands of eons. It is the same Nature that has been deified and worshipped in numerous forms. It is the same Nature whose First Law has been ignored and violated at every step by arrogant humanity.

Today humankind lives under the complete sway of fire which has transformed this Earth into a hell. That fire has donned the mask of a beautiful flower and placed itself at the center of the dinner table. Its enrapturing fragrance has been breathed into the very fiber of the entire human species.

The "civilized" human of today ridicules the idolatry of bygone ages, but nobody realizes that the masses now are the most extreme idolaters of all time. In former times people set up images of various animals and adored them; today they slaughter those animals and worship their charred carcasses.

The "civilized" human of today cannot fathom the barbarism under which the whole world lives at the present time. The "delicate," "refined," and "cultured" individual, who faints at the sight of a few drops of blood, calmly places on the dinner table the bloody heart, liver, or breast of a lamb and consumes it unabashedly. Had s/he seen from their childhood the slaughter and gore which tore that lamb away from its mother and killed it, there is no way s/he, or anybody else, would have eaten it. Such is the power of addiction; and it grows stronger the more one is removed from its true ramifications.

It is but one small step from the consumption of cooked lamb to cooked human. The only difference is that humanity is accustomed to one and not the other.

Cooked food is poison.

Chapter 40

Conclusions

"Must we then speak of this subject also;
and shall we write concerning things that are
not to be told, and shall we publish things not to
be divulged, and secrets not to be spoken aloud?"
— Julian, Emperor of Rome (361-363)

So long as human beings persist in consuming cooked food, there can be neither real civilization nor lasting health on Earth. At present, humankind is far from being civilized.

In a world that has fallen to this present standard and utter blindness, where disease is the norm, you may find it difficult to picture the enormous benefits that humanity will derive from raw-foodism. Almost instantaneously every disease will be swept away forever, and every addiction and crime against Nature will disappear from the face of the Earth. At the same time the expectation of life will increase two or three times. There will be an economic advance of such magnitude as would never before have been within human reach; as opposed to the situation now when all your government has to do is keep the economy somehow gasping and wheezing along so that the masses can be conditioned to accept any outrage.

These assertions are facts and not fiction, and, what is more, all those benefits can be procured in a very simple way. All one has to do is respect the most elementary Laws of Nature and prevent the destruction of the living and integral wheat. If one had the mental presence to penetrate and perceive the difference between the living, active wheat and the incinerated bread, one could easily deduce the difference between the organism of a raw-foodist and that of a cooked-foodist.

To all cooked-foodists war is peace, freedom is slavery, and ignorance is strength.

Closing one's eyes to basic truths and pretending that one can nurture one's self on dead, cooked proteins; they call this strength.

Freedom from disease, addiction, and civilization — the discipline of adhering to just raw foods — that is considered slavery.

People are indoctrinated and forced to adhere to the most unnatural laws. They are fed the cooked remains of enslaved, poisoned animals. They participate in the unchecked "development" of the land by concrete and buildings and live in artificial caves. This entire war against Nature is considered peace. In a state of war, people behave too naturally — of course that is intolerable to the "civilized." Let us just say that the only way you can have peace on Earth is to destroy every life form on the planet. Conflict is essential to life. If you want peace, go to the moon. How unfortunate it is that most wars are waged for the most unnatural reasons.

There can only be two reasons for rejecting the principles of raw-foodism:

1. Lack of common sense or instinct.

2. Complete absence of will-power and/or will-to-power.

All other reasons are mere pretexts, euphemized to cover up these two shortcomings.

Those who have been practicing one hundred percent raw-eating for three months would never agree to return to their abnormal mode of living. People who value their family's health will make that "experiment" of three months without a moment's hesitation.

Let us now look at the attitude adopted by the present rulers of the world and by other responsible authorities towards these vital problems. A letter we received from your First Lady Hillary Clinton showed us that she is in general sympathy with our views. In fact, we have not heard a single discordant voice from any quarter.

But this is not enough. In the United States, the activities of the FDA (a.k.a. - CFPA - Cooked Food and Poison Administration) and the USDA (a.k.a. - United States Department of Animal-abuse) have continued unabated. These abominable governing authorities knowingly condone and recommend the consumption of vast numbers of unnatural substances. Their activities are the worst thing since sliced bread.

We declare to all people and authoritative bodies that our publication is not just an interesting book to be read once and placed aside. It is a volume in which the most momentous and urgent problems of our time are discussed. It must be referenced again and again. Every sentence of it must be carefully weighed and considered for hours.

It would be a mistake if those rulers of the world were to treat raw-foodism as just one more routine question and, like all their other political and economic problems, submit it to bureaucrats for further study and consideration. For thousands of years there have been numerous experiments and studies, but they have all failed miserably. Today it is the absolute duty of the authorities to direct people to put an end to those destructive experiments and to return to a normal way of life. Today every sensible person is an expert in determining the difference between the natural and the unnatural, between the living and the lifeless. And the rulers of the world should be no different.

By the procrastination of this question the presidents, monarchs, premiers, and racial leaders will only harm themselves. While the so-called "experts" are busy examining the question, their own precious lives will be slipping through their fingers. Because of their advanced age most of them are already standing on the brink of the precipice. If by a bold decision they pull themselves away to safety, they will undoubtedly gain a healthy and happy life of forty to fifty years, an additional life in itself.

The great national leaders of the past attained their exalted positions by virtue of their capability, charisma, perseverance, and wisdom. Endowed with these qualities, they could have digested the principles of raw-foodism quickly and put them into practice with comparative ease. Any true leader has the ability to rule over their own person. What successes they could have achieved by inspiring their subjects by example remains unknown. Indeed, the destiny of any race or nation led by a raw-foodist is unfathomable.

Self-confident people in responsible positions should not give anyone the impression that they lack raw courage. Those leaders who are interested in the happiness and welfare of their peoples must plant the seeds of prosperity by their own personal examples. This will be the most useful and meritorious service to their people.

If one raw leader were to emerge in this world of slavery and mediocrity this Earth could be turned into a veritable paradise. What this world needs is decision and strength, not more lethargic democracy and bureaucratic committees.

During the last ten years a considerable amount of information has been received from every corner of the globe on the successes achieved by raw-foodism. This information demonstrates that there are thousands of convinced raw-foodists dispersed throughout the world, many of whom have been completely cured of serious diseases and are now leading the happiest of lives. These people are neither experts nor scientists. They are merely educated and intelligent individuals who have been able to comprehend the principles of raw-eating by their own insight and judgment, and have had the courage to make the necessary decisions.

Fortunately, the spread of our information and publications has been greatly facilitated by advances in communications and computer technology. Via the "information superhighway" we now have the ability to reach a global audience.

We hereby appeal to all intelligent people and future-oriented organizations for their assistance. Let them give us all the help they can in the dissemination of our publications. They can order twenty, fifty, or a hundred copies of our book and distribute them at their own discretion. Every book can save a life, cure a serious disease, or create the prospect of a blossoming future for a young child. At the present time there is no activity of greater value than that.

If we had the benefit of such a book ten years ago, today our relatives, friends, and pets would still be alive. If we had not been enlightened by our own rigorous search, we might not even be alive right now. Almost every single person on the planet is in the same condition and needs this information. It is necessary to familiarize them with the correct principles of nutrition as soon as possible.

Today we see how certain religious organizations spend enormous sums of money to distribute canned "goods" and other "non-perishable" items (whatever that means) to the poor and refined flour, rice, cow's milk, and various soups to entire nations. By distributing such unnatural and extremely degenerated foods to these people, they unwittingly commit a most grievous sin and violate the laws of their beloved god. What is it they fear about feeding those people the living potato or corn?

The time has come for the representatives of all religions to condemn decisively and unequivocally the degeneration of food by heating. Perhaps the very principles of raw-foodism might eradicate the very basis of their religions. These are the ideas you must ponder.

There was time when people thought that the Earth was stationary, while the Sun, planets, and stars went around it. If anybody expressed a contrary view, they were assumed, by short-sighted people, to be insane. The myopic masses could see with their own eyes that the Earth was fixed in its place while the Sun moved across the sky. It took only one scientific distinction and a few great scientists to awaken the minds of people throughout the world.

Precisely the same mentality prevails today. Humans apparently feel that raw plant foods, such as cabbage or cucumbers, may do them harm. Whereas they believe that wheat bread and brown rice, being "easily" digestible, "regulate" the functions of the stomach. They do not realize that it is the use of that bread and rice which is the real cause of a weak stomach, and that it is cabbage and cucumbers that will cure them in the long run.

Today, all of humanity is convinced that as soon as a sandwich is eaten, the regular requirements of the organism are satisfied. People are not aware that the cells struggle for nutrients and they remain quite hungry.

Today, all of humanity is convinced that in order to lead a healthy life one must be guided by various scientific calculations obtained in research laboratories. They are not aware that those calculations are completely false and harmful representations of the true picture.

Today, when people become ill, they are convinced that some drug or poison will cure them. They are not aware that drug therapy is more savage than blood-letting. No poison can ever perform a useful function.

They are not aware that all diseases have two causes: the continuous starvation of the normal cells due to a lack of raw nourishment and the pernicious effects of unnatural food extracts trapped within the organism. There is only one sensible way to free yourself from diseases once and for all. You must totally abstain from unnatural foods and drugs, and satisfy the needs of your cells by natural nutrition alone.

Drugs, which are commonly regarded as a means of curing diseases, are, in reality, the causes of diseases. It is a tragic mistake to search for any curative properties in a synthetic substance or an individual nutriment. Yet this is the very mistake humans have been making for thousands of years. There do not exist any curative substances in the world. There exist only the special factors that cause disease; once they are removed, diseases are automatically eradicated. Those factors are cooked, dead, and denatured food and the poisons which are misnamed "medicines."

People of today are proud of their civilization, but they are far from being really civilized. Real civilization should be measured not by mere technological progress, but by the ennoblement of the individual, the conquest of vices and addictions, the emancipation of the human intellect from superstitions, and the forwarding of a genetically pure population.

In order to gratify abnormal desires for food, humans burn eighty percent or more of the natural foods they place over the fire and bring about their own destruction by creating diseases artificially. The representatives of science, dismissing all emotional feelings, unscrupulously exploit the sacred name of science to further their own niggardly interests. In doing so they plunder people in a most ruthless manner.

Let those who continually discourse upon civilization prove that they themselves are civilized enough to comprehend the most elementary Laws of Nature. Only then will they understand the way to free humanity from pollution, confusion, and disease. It is amazing how hard people will work to achieve success, happiness, and comfort. Nobody realizes that you can have all these things instantly, simply by controlling what you put in your mouth. Only one distinction is required to double the life expectancy and quadruple the standard of living while preserving the planet for future generations.

Raw-foodism is the absolute command of Nature. You have seen the utter chaos and destruction caused by the infringement of the Laws of Nature. The entire life process of the Earth has been put in jeopardy by the consumption of unnatural substances. Natural nutrition is raw. It always has been; it always will be. That we should even have to prove that raw-foodism is the only normal and natural way to live is proof positive of the mental and moral perversity of this age. Cooked food *is* dead. Human evolution stopped when the first morsel of denatured food was consumed. Nothing unnatural can last for long. The forthcoming of raw-foodism, at this time, is the greatest event in the history of the world. The majesty and glory of raw-foodism imbues humanity with a new life. It is a beacon of light in a long, dark tunnel. It is the one way; it is the one Truth.

Cooked food is poison.

Raw is Nature's First Law.

All else is error.

Nature's Second Law will be unleashed upon the masses when circumstances demand it.

Appendix A

The Principles Of A
Raw-Food Transition & Lifestyle

1. The most important requisite for becoming a raw-foodist is a powerful, undiminished belief that raw nutrition is indeed the only normal and natural way to live. This belief must be the product of one's own conclusions. This underlying philosophy must be strong enough to carry you through the cyclical lows of the detoxification process. Chance, destiny, and fate cannot circumvent, hinder, or control the firm resolve of the determined.

2. Concerning will-power & diet: To be successful in anything, it does not matter what, you must be willing to take a step outside of your comfort zone. All successful people have this in common. You will realize your comfort zone was never really comfortable.

3. Decisively cut off the negative influences of mass media, by refusing to watch television, listen to the radio, read the newspaper, etc. Additionally, reevaluate and choose your associations carefully. Weed out negativity. Remember, you become the sum total of the six people you associate with most.

*"Without doubt, the most common weakness of all
human beings is the habit of leaving their minds
open to the negative influence of other people."*
— **Napoleon Hill**

4. Eating seasonal fruits and vegetables is Nature's way of telling you what to eat and when.

5. For ideal digestion and assimilation, eat one food at a time. Maintain a mono-diet. You would not find a pineapple tree next to an orange tree, next to an apple tree, next to a grape vine, next to a watermelon patch; that's why you should never eat a fruit salad. Also, what are the repercussions of eating fruits from a grocery store that have been imported from all around the globe? An orange from Florida, an apple from Washington, an avocado from San Diego, a pineapple from Hawaii, a banana from Ecuador. (Though we stress a mono-diet, we do distribute raw-recipes. Please contact our organization through the information provided at the end of this book).

6. Eating lunch at 12 o'clock noon every day is one of the most ridiculous customs ever practiced. It is like filling your car up with 10 gallons of gasoline every day, at 12 noon, no matter how empty or full the gas tank is. A truly free individual does not follow rules and dead traditions. Truly free people never regulate their conduct by hypnotic suggestion or the false dicta of others, for when they do, they are no longer free.

7. It is a common myth that food is the only thing that gives you energy. If this was true, you could lay in bed all day and eat raw foods and be healthy, right? Wrong. The body also needs sun and air. The best source for energy is, in fact, air. Deep-breathing actually diminishes the body's need for food. There are accounts of people living high in the mountains that subsist exclusively on air and a little snow.

8. Fast one day a week: an auspicious and natural way to start with the cleansing activity.

9. The nutrition by race approach: Humans are fruitarian by nature and design. But the percentage of vegetables, herbs, sprouts, roots, and other natural foods within the diet may vary

from 5% to 50% depending on the racial background of the person and their present environment. Generally:

a. Tropical races and climates are conducive to 95 to 100% fruitarianism.

b. Sub-tropical races and climates are conducive to 80 to 95% fruitarianism.

c. As one continues southward/northward away from the equator or into more extreme climes (mountains or desert) the races and climates become conducive to up to 50% non-fruit foods in the diet. d. The northern races may have more tolerance for raw meat. Though eating raw meat is unnatural for the human organism, for cooked meat-addicts, the consumption of small amounts of raw meat may ease the transitional period to a raw-food diet.

10. Artificial cooling is just as unnatural as artificial heating — though perhaps not as harmful. Refrigeration is unnatural.

11. People always ask us if a certain thing is okay to eat (sprouted bread, pickles, bottled juice, etc.). The best way to determine this is to put the foodstuff in your hand and ask yourself, "Does this exist in Nature in this exact state?" If yes, it's okay. If not, it's been denatured and you are tampering with Nature and your health.

12. To deflect criticism, make a game out of situations where people ask you why you eat the way you do.

Appendix B

The Land Mammals

Is a human being a carnivore, herbivore, or omnivore?			
	CARNIVORE	**HERBIVORE**	**HUMAN**
1	Teeth are long, sharp, and pointed. No flat molar teeth. Sharp canine teeth.	Front and canine teeth may be sharp or pointed. Back teeth are flattened for grinding.	All teeth are flattened, especially the back molars. Dullest canine teeth of all primates.
2	To facilitate tearing and biting, jaw is moving up and down (vertically).	To facilitate the grinding of vegetable foods, jaw can move both up and down (vertically) and side side (horizontally).	To facilitate the grinding of vegetable foods, jaw can move both up and down (vertically) and side side (horizontally).
3	No lip or pouchy cheek structure.	Adaptable lip pouchy cheek structure.	Refined lip and pouchy cheek structure.
4	Shape of the face allows the carnivore to dig into a carcass and rip out the entrails.	Shape of the face allows the animal to pull vegetation off of plants.	Shape of the face clearly indicates that humans have no ability to rip out entrails with their mouth.
5	Forward facing eyes; binocular vision.	**Herbivores with predators:** radial eyeset allowing for wide field of vision. **Herbivores without predators:** forward facing eyes; binocular vision.	Forward facing eyes; binocular vision. Humans have no natural predators.
6	Drinks water by lifting it into the throat by the tongue.	Drinks water by suction.	Drinks water by suction.

	CARNIVORE	HERBIVORE	HUMAN
7	Tongue is rough and thin.	Tongue is smooth and thick to manipulate vegetable matter into the back molars for grinding.	Tongue is smooth and thick to manipulate vegetable matter into the back molars for grinding.
8	Stomach is a round sack that secretes 10 to 20 times as much acid as a herbivore.	Stomach is oblong and complex; stomach acid is 10 to 20 times weaker than a carnivore's.	Stomach is oblong and complex; stomach acid is 10 to 20 times weaker than a carnivore's.
9	Intestines are 3 times as long as the trunk of the body; their design facilitates rapid expulsion of fleshy matter.	Intestines are at least 8 to 12 times as long as the trunk of the body; they are designed for extracting all nutrients from plant fiber.	Intestines are at least 12 times as long as the trunk, and an integral part of the most sophisticated juice extractor in the world: the human digestive system.
10	Liver contains uricase, an enzyme used to break down uric acid; it can eliminate 10 to 15 times as much uric acid as a herbivore's liver.	Liver has a low tolerance for uric acid.	Liver has a low tolerance for uric acid.
11	Bowels are smooth and short for quick expulsion.	Bowels are sucified and complex for the reconstitution of waste matter.	Bowel walls are puckered, convoluted, and full of deep pouches for the reconstitution of waste matter.
12	Digestive system has the capacity to expel large amounts of foreign cholesterol.	Digestive system has no capacity to expel foreign cholesterol.	Digestive system has no capacity to expel foreign cholesterol.
13	Saliva is acidic.	Saliva is alkaline; it contains enzymes specifically designed to break down starchy carbohydrates.	Saliva is alkaline; it contains ptyalin, an enzyme that specifically designed to break down starchy carbohydrates.
14	Blood is acidic.	Blood is alkaline.	Blood is alkaline.
15	Urine is acidic.	Urine is alkaline.	Urine is alkaline.
16	Cools itself primarily through action of the tongue and mouth.	Cools itself primarily through perspiration.	Cools itself primarily through perspiration.

	CARNIVORE	HERBIVORE	HUMAN
17	All four feet are clawed (to rip into flesh).	All four feet are hoofed (cloven), or hands and feet contain individual digits (fingers or toes) with nails.	Hands and feet contain individual digits with nails and opposable thumbs. Hands are perfectly designed to reach out, grab fruit, and peel it.

Conclusion: The human is the most herbivorious of the herbivores: a frugivore.

Appendix C

Studies And Experiments

1. F.M. Pottenger conducted a 10 year study on the effects of heated, processed foods on the facial dental structure of animals which was first published in the *American Journal of Orthodontics and Oral Surgery*. It is, to date, the most extensive study done on the effect of a cooked-food diet on an animal's life cycle. Under the most rigorous standards of his day, Pottenger raised a colony of 900 cats placed on controlled diets. Only meat and milk were used and were given either in their raw or cooked state. The cats fed on raw food produced healthy kittens year after year. The cats fed the cooked version of the exact same food developed the same diseases which afflict human populations. These diseases included: cancer, osteoporosis, heart disease, glandular malfunctioning, kidney disease, sexual impotency, paralysis, pneumonia, arthritis, difficulty in labor, severe irritability (making the cats difficult to handle). The first generation of kittens born to the cooked-food cats were ill and abnormal. The second generation were born either already diseased or dead. By the third generation, the mothers were sterile. His startling discovery: Inherited damage created by eating cooked foods requires four generations of animals nourished on raw foods to correct.

The excrement from the cooked-food cats was so toxic that the plants fertilized with it were stunted and weak; whereas the plants grown in soil fertilized by the excrement of the raw-food cats grew normally. Implication: Cooked food disrupts the entire life-cycle.

Dr. Pottenger conducted similar tests on white mice. His results were identical to those in the cat experiment.

2. Dr. Weston Price, an American dentist, spent 20 years (1920-1940) traveling the world to study "primitive" societies. He examined the dietary patterns of these societies. The average "primitive" diet consisted of simple, fresh, and largely uncooked foods which were typically gathered and eaten immediately. He compared this diet to the teeth and bone development, the incidence of dental caries, and the overall physical and mental health of those "primitive" peoples. He found that health is directly related to the wholeness and freshness of the foods people consume. He recounted his findings, complete with photographs and statistics, in his famous book *Nutrition and Physical Degeneration,* published in 1945. His main conclusion: Processed foods create appalling problems for human health.

3. Dr. Paul Kouchakoff, at the Institute of Clinical Chemistry in Sausanne, Switzerland in 1930, reported that the consumption of raw plant foods does not change the chemical make-up of the blood. However, when cooked food is consumed, augmentation of white blood cells occurs. Translation: The human body fights cooked food like a disease or the white blood cells are actually the mutagenic products of cooked food.

4. Lewis E. Cook Jr. and Junko Yasui recounted a powerful study in their book *Goldot*. The experiment involved three groups of rats.

The first group of rats were fed, from birth, diets of raw fruits, vegetables, nuts, and whole grains. They grew into completely healthy specimens and never suffered from any diseases. They grew rapidly, never became fat, reproduced with vigor and enthusiasm, and had healthy offspring. They were always playful and affectionate. Upon reaching an age equivalent to 80 human years they were put to death and autopsied. All their organs, glands, and tissues appeared in perfect condition without any signs of aging or degeneration.

The second group of rats were fed, from birth, diets of cooked foods including: white bread, meat, milk, salt, soda, candy, cakes, vitamins, medicines, etc. These rats became fat and were afflicted by the very same diseases that afflict present-day society including: colds, fevers, pneumonia, poor eyesight, cataracts, heart disease, arthritis, cancer, etc.

During the life-cycle of the second group, the rats exhibited vicious, nervous, and self-destructive behavior. They had to be separated to keep them from killing each other. Their offspring were consistently ill and displayed the same behavioral characteristics as their parents.

Most of the second group died prematurely from diseases or various epidemics which swept through the colony. Autopsies performed on this group revealed extensive degeneration in all the organs, glands, and tissues of their bodies

The third group of rats were fed a diet identical to the second group until they reached an equivalent human age of 40 years. They displayed the same symptoms of ill-health and self-destructive behavior as the second group.

At the end of this time period, the rats were placed on a strict water fast for several days. Then they were fed the raw diet of the first group. This diet was alternated with periods of fasting. Within one month, their health and behavioral patterns changed dramatically. They became affectionate, playful, and never became ill. Autopsies performed after the equivalent of 80 human years indicated this group had reversed its degenerative tissue damage.

Conclusion: It is never too late to revitalize an animal organism through natural nutrition.

5. In India, Sir Robert McCarrison fed monkeys their usual diet, but in a cooked form. All the monkeys developed severe intestinal problems. The autopsies revealed gastric and intestinal ulcers. Conclusion: Cooked food kills.

6. In Switzerland, O. Stiner fed guinea pigs their usual diet, but in a cooked form. His animals succumbed to numerous diseases in including: anemia, scurvy, goiter, dental caries, glandular degeneration, and (when ten cc of pasteurized milk was added to their diet) arthritis.

7. A study appeared in the *British Medical Journal* (Vol. 14, No. 10) in 1960 which clearly exposed the dangers of pasteurization. The study was entitled "The Effect of Heat Treatment on the Nutritive Value of Milk for the Young Calf: The Effect of Ultra-High Temperature Treatment and of Pasteurization." It entailed feeding calves their mother's milk after it had been cooked. The calves fed on pasteurized milk died before maturity in nine out of ten cases. Conclusion: Cooked milk is poison even for the animal it was designed for.

8. A study of rats, whose tooth decay patterns are virtually identical to human teeth, appeared in the *Southern California Dental Association Journal* (Vol. 31, No. 9) in 1963. The rats were divided into three groups. The first group received a standard, cooked rat-food — they averaged less than one cavity per rat. The second group was fed a diet heavy in refined sugar — they averaged five and one half cavities per rat. The third group was fed pasteurized milk — they averaged nine and one half cavities per rat. Conclusion: Contrary to popular belief, pasteurized milk does not strengthen the bones and teeth but significantly weakens them.

9. Food toxicologist, Leonard Bjeldanes, and his fellow researchers at the University of California at Berkeley, discovered that cooked eggs and cattle muscle (beef) contained substances which caused genetic mutations in bacteria. The longer and hotter that these foods were cooked, the greater the mutagenic activity of the bacteria. Frying and grilling being the most dangerous, roasting and baking less so.

10. In 1935, Clive McCay at Cornell University demonstrated that when mammals are underfed from weaning, their lifespans were increased considerably. His complete works are recounted in his book *Notes on the History of Nutrition Research* published in 1973.

11. In 1979, Roy Walford and Richard Weindruch began studies which eventually proved that adult animals reach signifi-

cantly higher ages if they are consistently underfed. Some of their mice lived 40 percent longer than those fed a "complete" diet. Some of their fish lived three times the normal age for their species. Of the control group of mice fed a "complete" diet, 50 percent of the animals ultimately developed cancer. Of the group fed a restricted diet, 13 percent ultimately developed cancer, and did so much later in life. Their research also indicated that underfed animals stay physiologically younger for longer.

12. Russell Chittendon, professor of physiology at Yale University, recounted in his book *The Nutrition of Men* (1907), his experiments on three groups of people: athletes, moderately-active workers, and university professors. Each was fed a varied diet, which included cooked-meat dishes. His main goal was to determine to what extent protein was essential for health, energy, and stamina. Not only did his experimental subjects report feeling better and stronger as their fruit and vegetable consumption increased, but experiments on their fitness clearly indicated that the fitness of all three groups improved when they ate fewer calories and less than half their normal protein intake. Conclusion: a fleshy protein intake decreases health, endurance, and stamina.

Fascinated by his research, Chittendon adopted a vegetarian diet and quickly rid himself of a rheumatic knee-joint problem, periodic headaches, and a digestive disorder.

13. From his work with prescribing raw foods to patients, Dr. John Douglass found that common addictions (alcohol and cigarettes) seem to lose their potency on a diet of raw foods. Will-power did not seem to play a part. Experimenting with specific raw foods and their effects, he found that some, such as sunflower seeds, were particularly effective at combating addictive cravings. His conclusion: Raw foods sensitize the body to what is good for it and what is bad for it. Some of his findings were discussed in an article entitled "Nutrition, Nonthermally-prepared Food and Nature's Message to Man" which appeared in the *Journal of the International Academy of Preventative*

Medicine (Vol. VII, No. 2) in July of 1982.

14. In the 1930s Professor Karl Eimer, the director of the Medical Clinic at the University of Vienna tested the effects of a 100 percent raw-food diet on athletes. He placed several of the top athletes in his country on a program of high-intensity physical training. This would continue for two weeks and then suddenly, without any transition, he would place them upon an entirely raw diet. Without any exception the athletes experienced faster reflexes, more flexibility, and improved stamina. He discussed his work in an article (written in German) entitled *Klinik Schwenkenhacher,* printed in the July 1933 edition of *Zeitschrift fur Ernahrung.*

In 1938, Dr. Eimer's colleague and the chief doctor at the University of Vienna, Professor Hans Eppinger showed that raw nutrition increases cellular respiration and efficiency.

Caveats:

A. The reason scientists do experiments on animals is because cooked-food addiction has clouded everyone's mind. They cannot think for themselves. They cannot see reality, so they need their proof demonstrated to them by torturing defenseless creatures.

B. Any study or experiment, in which the subject is a cooked-food human or animal, cannot be precisely accurate in any way because the entire organism has been weakened and corrupted.

There are countless studies in the world to support the philosophy of nutrition, but the most profound study is that which one performs on her/his own body. What is amazing about this philosophy is that you can prove it conclusively true by your own experience.

Appendix D

Vegetarian Diet vs. Meat-Centered
Diet Facts & Statistics (1996)

If you still are not convinced of the absolute benefits of The Raw-Food Diet and the utter suicide of being a cooked-foodist, we have included an extensive list of facts and statistics called "Realities," most of which was originally compiled by John Robbins and revised and updated by Nature's First Law. Though most of these facts simply compare a vegetarian diet to an animal-based diet, remember that the differences between the two, however great, are much greater still when one compares the differences between a raw-food diet and a vegetarian or vegan diet.

Humans and Livestock

1. Human population of the United States: @ 300 million
2. Number of humans that can be fed by the grain and soybeans eaten by U.S. livestock: 1.4 billion
3. Percentage of corn grown in U.S. eaten by livestock: 85%; percentage of corn eaten by humans: 15% (99.999% of which is cooked)
4. Percentage of oats grown in U.S. eaten by livestock: 95%
5. Percentage of protein wasted by cycling grain through livestock: 90%
6. Percentage of carbohydrate wasted by cycling grain through livestock: 99%
7. Percentage of dietary fiber wasted by cycling grain through livestock: 100%
8. How frequently a child dies of starvation: Every 2 seconds

9. Amount of potatoes that can be grown on 1 acre (4,047 square meters) of land: 20,000 lbs. (9,072 kg)

10. Amount of beef that can be grown on 1 acre (4,047 square meters) of land: 165 lbs. (75 kg)

11. Percentage of U.S. agricultural land used to produce beef: 56%

12. Amount of grain and soybeans needed to produce 1 pound (or kilogram) of feedlot beef: 16 lbs. (7.3 kg)

13. Amount of protein fed to chickens to produce 1 pound (or kilogram) of protein as chicken flesh: 5 lbs. (2.3 kg)

14. Amount of protein fed to hogs to produce 1 pound (or kilogram) of protein as hog flesh: 7.5 lbs. (3.4 kg)

15. Number of children who starve to death every day: 40,000

16. Number of pure vegetarians who can be fed on the amount of land needed to feed 1 person consuming meat-based diet: 20 (This number could be closer to 150 if you're talking about pure raw-vegetarians.)

17. Number of people who will starve to death this year: 60,000,000

18. Number of people who could be adequately fed by the grain saved if Americans reduced their intake of meat by 10%: 60,000,000

Soil

19. Historic cause of demise of many great civilizations: Topsoil depletion

20. Percentage of original U.S. topsoil lost to date: 75%

21. Amount of U.S. cropland lost each year to soil erosion: 4 million acres (16,187 square kilometers, or size of Connecticut)

22. Percentage of U.S. topsoil loss directly associated with livestock raising: 85%

Trees

23. Amount of U.S forest which has been cleared to create cropland to produce a meat-centered diet: 260 million acres (1.05 million square kilometers)

24. How often an acre (4,047 square meters) of U.S. trees disappears: Every 8 seconds

25. Amount of trees spared per year by each individual who switches to a pure vegetarian diet: 1 acre (4,047 square meters)

Rainforests

26. A driving force behind the destruction of the tropical rainforests: American meat habit

27. Amount of meat imported annually by U.S. from Costa Rica, El Salvador, Guatemala, Nicaragua, Honduras, and Panama: Less than the average house cat

28. Current rate of species extinction due to destruction of tropical rainforests and related habitats: 1000 per year

Water

29. User of more than half of all water used for all purposes in the United States: Livestock production

30. The quantity of water used in the production of the average cow: Sufficient to float a destroyer

31. Water needed to produce 1 pound (0.45 kg) of wheat: 25 gallons (95 liters)

32. Water needed to produce 1 pound (0.45 kg) of meat: 2,500 gallons (9,465 liters)

33. Cost of common hamburger meat if water used by meat industry was not subsidized by U.S. taxpayers: $35 per pound ($77 per kg)

34. Current cost for 1 pound (0.45 kg) of protein from wheat: $1.50

35. Current cost for 1 pound (0.45 kg) of protein from beefsteak: $15.40

36. Cost for 1 pound (0.45 kg) of protein from beefsteak if U.S. taxpayers ceased subsidizing meat industry's use of water: $89

Petroleum and Energy

37. Length of time world's petroleum reserves would last (with current technologies) if all human beings ate meat-centered diet: 13 years

38. Length of time world's petroleum reserves would last (with current technologies) if all human beings ate vegetarian diet: 260 years

39. Principal reason for U.S. intervention in Persian Gulf: Dependence on foreign oil

40. Barrels of oil imported daily by U.S.: 6.8 million

41. Percentage of energy return (as food energy per fossil energy expended) of most energy efficient farming of meat: 34.5%

42. Percentage of energy return (as food energy per fossil energy expended) of least energy efficient plant food: 328%

43. Amount of soy beans produced by the amount of fossil fuel needed to produce 1 pound (0.45 kg) of feedlot beef: 40 lbs. (18.1 kg)

44. Percentage of raw materials consumed in U.S. for all purposes presently consumed to produce current meat-centered diet: 33%

45. Percentage of raw materials consumed in U.S. for all purposes needed to produce pure vegetarian diet: 2%

Sewage Systems

46. Production of excrement by total U.S. population: 12,000 lbs. (5443 kg) per second

47. Production of excrement by U.S. livestock: 250,000 lbs. (113,400 kg) per second

48. Sewage systems in U.S. cities: Common

49. Sewage systems in U.S. feedlots: Nil

50. Amount of waste produced annually by U.S. livestock in confinement operations which is not recycled: 1 billion tons (907 billion kg)

51. Relative concentration of feedlot wastes compared to raw domestic sewage: Ten to several hundred times more highly concentrated

52. Where feedlot waste typically ends up: Human water supply

Medical School Nutritional Training

53. Number of U.S. medical schools: 125

54. Number of U.S. medical schools with a required course in nutrition: 30

55. Training in nutrition received during 4 years of medical school by the average U.S. physician: 2.5 hours

Heart Attacks

56. How frequently a heart attack strikes in the U.S.: Every 25 seconds

57. How frequently a heart attack kills in the U.S.: Every 45 seconds

58. Most common cause of death in U.S.: Heart attack

59. Risk of death from heart attack by average American man: 50%

60. Risk of death from heart attack by average American purely vegetarian man: 4%

61. Risk of death from heart attack by average American raw-foodist: 0%

62. Amount you reduce your risk of heart attack by reducing your consumption of meat, dairy products and eggs 10%: 9%

63. Amount you reduce your risk of heart attack by reducing your consumption of meat, dairy products and eggs 50%: 45%

64. Amount you reduce your risk of heart attack by reducing your consumption of meat, dairy products and eggs 100%: 90%

65. Rise in blood cholesterol from consuming 1 egg per day: 12%

66. Rise in heart attack risk from 12% rise in blood cholesterol: 24%

Meat, Dairy, and Egg Industries

67. Meat, dairy, and egg industries claim there is no reason to be concerned about your blood cholesterol as long as it is: "Normal"

68. Risk of dying of a disease caused by clogged arteries (atherosclerosis) if your blood cholesterol is "normal": Over 50%

69. Risk of dying of a disease caused by clogged arteries (atherosclerosis) if you do not consume saturated fat and cholesterol: 5%

70. Leading sources of saturated fat and cholesterol in American diets: Meat, dairy products, and eggs

71. World populations with high meat intakes who do not have correspondingly high rates of colon cancer: None

72. World populations with low meat intakes who do not have correspondingly low rates of colon cancer: None

73. Increased risk of breast cancer for women who eat meat daily compared to women who eat meat less than once a week: 4 times higher

74. Egg Board's advertising slogan: "The incredible, edible egg"

75. Increased risk of breast cancer for women who eat eggs daily compared to women who eat eggs less than once a week: 3 times higher

76. Milk producer's original advertising campaign slogan: "Everyone needs milk"

77. What the Federal Trade Commission called the "Everyone needs milk" slogan: "False, misleading and deceptive"

78. Milk producer's revised campaign slogans: "Milk has something for everybody," and "Milk does a body good"

79. Increased risk of breast cancer for women who eat butter and cheese 3 or more times a week compared to women who eat these foods less than once a week: 3 times higher

80. Part of female chicken's body that produces eggs: Ovaries

81. Increased risk of fatal ovarian cancer for women who eat eggs 3 or more times a week compared to women who eat eggs less than once a week: 3 times higher

82. Food males in the U.S. are conditioned to think of as "manly": Animal products (mostly meat)

83. Increased risk of fatal prostate cancer for men who consume meats, cheese, milk and eggs daily compared to men who eat these foods sparingly or not at all: 3.6 times higher

84. The Meat Board tells you: "Today's meats are low in fat"

85. The Meat Board shows you: A serving of beef they claim has "only 300 calories"

86. The Meat Board does not tell you: The serving of beef they show you is only 3 ounces (85 grams), which is half the size of an average serving of beef, and has been surgically de-fatted with a scalpel

87. The dairy industry tells you: Whole milk is 3.5% fat

88. The dairy industry does not tell you: That 3.5% figure is based on weight and most of the weight in milk is water

89. The dairy industry does not want you to know: The amount of calories as fat in whole milk is 50%

90. The meat company Oscar Mayer tells you: It is a "myth" that hot dogs are fatty

91. Oscar Meyer demonstrates their point by comparing the fatness of hot dogs to such high-fat bastions as mayonnaise, margarine, salad dressing, and cream cheese

92. The Dairy Council tells you: Milk is Nature's most perfect food

93. The Dairy Council does not tell you: Milk is Nature's most perfect food for a baby calf, who has four stomachs, will double its weight in 47 days, and is destined to weigh 300 pounds (136 kg) within a year

94. The Dairy Council tells children to: Grow up big and strong and drink lots of milk

95. The Dairy Council occasionally tells children: The enzyme necessary for digestion of milk is lactase

96. The Dairy Council never tells children: 20% of Caucasian children and 80% of black children have no lactase in their intestines. (Humanity has gone so far as to create a pill that aids in the digestion of dairy products. This is just as insane as taking a pill before you drink motor oil to help in the digestion of that motor oil. If your body is not designed to naturally digest certain substance then maybe you should not consume it)

97. The meat, dairy and egg industries tell you: Animal products constitute 2 of the "Basic 4" food groups

98. The meat, dairy and egg industries do not tell you: There were originally 12 basic food groups, before these industries applied enormous political pressure on behalf of their products

99. The meat, dairy and egg industries tell you: You are well-fed only with animal products

100. The meat, dairy and egg industries do not tell you: The diseases which are commonly prevented, consistently improved, and even cured by a vegetarian diet include: Heart disease, strokes, osteoporosis, kidney stones, breast cancer, colon cancer, prostate cancer, pancreatic cancer, ovarian cancer, cervical cancer, stomach cancer, endometrial cancer, diabetes, hypoglycemia kidney disease, peptic ulcers, constipation, hemorrhoids, hiatal hernias, diverticulosis, obesity, gallstones, hypertension, asthma, irritable colon syndrome, salmonellosis, trichinosis, etc.

"We live in a crazy time, when people who make food choices that are healthy and compassionate are often considered weird, while people are considered normal whose eating habits promote disease and are dependent on enormous suffering."
— **John Robbins**

Pesticides in Livestock

101. Chlorinated hydrocarbon pesticide residues in the U.S. diet: Supplied by meat: 55%

102. Supplied by dairy products: 23%

103. Supplied by vegetables: 6%

104. Supplied by fruits: 4%

105. Supplied by grains: 1%

106. Percentage of U.S. mother's milk containing significant levels of DDT: 99%

107. Percentage of U.S. vegetarian mother's milk containing significant levels of DDT: 8%

108. Relative pesticide contamination in breast milk of meat-eating mothers compared to pesticide contamination in breast milk of vegetarian mothers: 35 times as high

109. Percentage of male college students sterile in 1950: 0.5%

110. Percentage of male college students sterile in 1978: 25%

111. Sperm count of average American male compared to 35 years ago: Down 30%

112. Principle reason for sterility and sperm count reduction of U.S. males: Chlorinated hydrocarbon pesticides (including dioxin, DDT, etc.)

113. Percentage of hydrocarbon pesticide residues in American diet attributable to meats, dairy products, fish, and eggs: 94%

114. The Meat Board tells you not to be concerned about the dioxins and other pesticides in today's beef because: The quantities are so small

115. The Meat Board does not want you to know: How potent dioxin and other pesticides are

116. The Meat Board particularly does not want you know: A mere ounce (28.4 grams) of dioxin could kill 10 million people

117. The United States Department of Agriculture (USDA) tells you: Your meat is inspected

118. The USDA does not tell you: Less than 1 out of every 250,000 slaughtered animals is tested for toxic chemical residues

119. The dye used for many years by the USDA to stamp meats "Choice," "Prime," or "U.S. No. 1 USDA": Violet Dye No. 1

120. Current status of Violet Dye No. 1: Banned as a proven carcinogen

"It is our alarming misfortune that so primitive
a science has armed itself with the most modern
terrible weapons, and that in turning them against
the insects it has also turned them against the Earth."
— **Rachel Carson**

Inhumane Treatment of Livestock

121. Wingspan of average leghorn chicken: 26 inches (66 cm)
122. Space average leghorn chicken is given in egg factories: 6 inches (15.3 cm)
123. Number of 700+ lb. (318+ kg) pigs confined to space the size of a twin bed in typical factory farm: 3
124. Reason today's veal is so tender: Calves are never allowed to take a single step
125. Reason today's veal is whitish-pink: Calves force-fed on anemia producing diet
126. McDonald's brags: Billions and billions sold
127. McDonald's does not brag about: Millions and millions butchered
128. McDonald's clown, Ronald McDonald, tells children: Hamburgers grow in hamburger patches and love to be eaten
129. McDonald's clown, Ronald McDonald, does not tell children: Hamburgers are ground up, cooked cows who have had their throats slit by machetes or their brains bashed in with sledgehammers
130. Original actor to play Ronald McDonald: Jeff Juliano
131. Diet now followed by Jeff Juliano: Vegetarian
132. Number of animals killed for meat per hour in the U.S.: 500,000
133. Occupation with highest turnover rate in the U.S.: Slaughterhouse worker
134. Cost to render an animal unconscious prior to slaughter with captive bolt pistol so that process in done humanely: $.01
135. Reason given by meat industry for not utilizing captive bolt pistol: Too expensive

"The greatness of a nation can be judged
by the way its animals are treated."
—Gandhi

Antibiotics in Livestock

136. Percentage of total antibiotics used in the U.S. fed routinely to livestock: 55%

137. Percentage of staphylococci infections resistant to penicillin in 1960: 13%

138. Percentage of staphylococci infections resistant to penicillin in 1988: 91%

139. Reason: Breeding of antibiotic resistant bacteria in factory farms due to routine feeding of antibiotics to livestock

140. Effectiveness of all "wonder-drug" antibiotics: Declining rapidly

141. Reason: Breeding of antibiotic resistant bacteria in factory farms due to routine feeding of antibiotics to livestock

142. Response by entire European Economic Community to routine feeding of antibiotics to livestock: Ban

143. Response by American meat and pharmaceutical industries to routine feeding of antibiotics to livestock: Full and complete support

Vegetarian Athletes

144. Only man to win Ironman Triathlon more than twice: Dave Scott (6 time winner)

145. Food choices of Dave Scott: Vegetarian

146. World record holder for 1 day triathlon (Swim 4.8 miles (7.7 km), cycle 185 miles (298 km), run 52.5 miles (84.5 km): Sixto Lenares

147. Food choices of Sixto Lenares: Strict vegetarian

148. Athlete who most totally dominated Olympic sport in track and field history: Edwin Moses (undefeated in 8 years, 400 meter hurdles)

149. Food choices of Edwin Moses: Vegetarian

150. Other notable vegetarian athletes:

- Stan Price (world record bench-press)
- Carl Lewis (world's fastest man, 8 Olympic gold medals, 7 world records)
- Robert Sweetgall (world's premier ultra-distance walker)
- Paavo Nurmi (20 world records in distance running, 9 Olympic medals)
- Bill Pickering (world record - swimming English Channel)
- Murray Rose (world records - swimming 400 and 1500 meter freestyles)
- Andreas Cahling (winner - Mr. International body-building championships)
- Roy Hilligan (winner - Mr. America body-building championships)
- Pierro Verot (world record for downhill endurance skiing)
- Estelle Gray and Cheryl Merek (world record for cross-country tandem cycling)
- James and Jonathan deDonato (world record for distance butterfly stroke swimming)
- Ridgely Abele (winner of 8 national championships in Karate, including U.S. Karate Association World Championships)
- Peter Burwash (highest fitness index of any athlete in Canada)
- Alan Jones (world record for continuous sit-ups - 17,003)

151. Raw-foodist athletes:

- George Allen (held the world record for walking from Land's End in Cornwall to John O'Groats at northern tip of Scotland; he lives mostly on raw vegetables)
- Barbara Moore (broke George Allen's walking record)
- Fausto Coppi and Luis Ocana (world-renowned cyclists trained on raw-foods by French herbalist Maurice Messegue)
- Dick Gregory (In 1974 he ran 900 miles (1450 kilometers) exclusively on fruit juice; a one-time American comedian, he is now a raw-food nutritionist who often works in the sport of boxing — he has worked with boxers such as heavyweight champion Riddick Bowe).
- Joe "The Atom" Greenstein (American strongman who enjoyed wide popularity in the 1930s; he was best known for pulling trains with his teeth)

> *"In sports, raw-foodists will establish*
> *new and unprecedented records.*
> *The age long dream of athletes*
> *is fulfilled by 100% raw-eating. "*
> — **Nature's First Law**

How much more obvious can it be? After knowing these facts, how can anyone believe that the consumption of animal products is not the most dangerous of addictions? Now that you have seen the differences between a meat-centered diet and a vegetarian diet, remember that the differences between a raw-foodist and a vegetarian (who may eat dairy products, bread, cooked vegetables, etc.) are far greater still.

How To Reach Nature's First Law

If you have any questions or comments about any of the material contained in this book, feel free to write, call, or E-mail Nature's First Law. We seek correspondence with all like-minded objective truth-seekers. However, please do not try to refute the Laws of Nature. That is not tolerated by our organization. You cannot put Nature on the stand. Further information concerning membership criteria (which are extremely strict), bulk book orders, other products, such as video and audio tapes, as well as special products for the true devotees of Nature's First Law, is also available.

Nature's First Law
P.O. Box 900202
San Diego, CA 92190 U.S.A.
(619) 645-7282
(800) 205-2350 - orders only

E-mail: nature@io-online.com
Internet Homepage: http://www.io-online.com/~nature